**Advance Praise for *The Myth of Aging***

"Dr. Gilberg has assembled a one-of-a kind, encyclopedic collection of information vital to mental and emotional health. *The Myth of Aging* is a groundbreaking, life-changing, must-read guide to living with purpose and passion. Never before has a book combined clinical insight with this much heart and soul."

—Los Angeles Tribune

## Also by Co-Author Jon Land

*No Surrender: Faith, Family, and Finding Your Way*

*1st and Forever: Making the Case for the Future of Football*

*Chasing the Dragon: How to Win the War on Drugs*

*Guardian: Life in the Crosshairs of the CIA's War on Terror*

*Overcoming: Lessons in Triumphing Over Adversity and the Power of Our Common Humanity*

*The Living Room: A Lung Cancer Community of Courage*

*Walking in the Mud: A Navy SEAL's 10 Rules for Surviving the New Normal*

*Justice Never Rests: A U.S. Attorney's Battle Against Murderers, Drug Lords, Mob Kingpins & Cults*

# THE MYTH OF AGING

A Prescription for Emotional and Physical Well-Being

**ARNOLD GILBERG MD**
**WITH JON LAND**

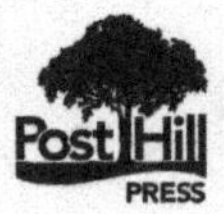

A POST HILL PRESS BOOK
ISBN: 979-8-89565-120-9
ISBN (eBook): 979-8-89565-121-6

The Myth of Aging:
A Prescription for Emotional and Physical Well-Being


Cover design by Cody Corcoran



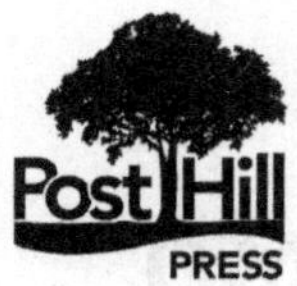


Post Hill Press
New York • Nashville
posthillpress.com

Published in the United States of America
1 2 3 4 5 6 7 8 9 10

To my wife, Gloria, for her unconditional love,
To my children and grandchildren for
teaching me how to live better,
And to my patients for letting me into their lives.

The mind and body are like parallel universes.
Anything that happens in the mental universe
must leave tracks in the physical one.

—Deepak Chopra

# TABLE OF CONTENTS

# PREFACE

I've been a practicing psychiatrist for more than fifty years, during which time I've seen more patients than I can count. But for every one of them I've helped, there's another thousand I could have. So I wrote *The Myth of Aging* to give me the opportunity to help those I couldn't see in a lifetime of office visits.

I've learned a lot over the years, and I want to share some of that knowledge with you. I want to help you improve your life or, at least, the parts of it that are holding you back or keeping you from being the best and happiest person you can be. I want people to have the tools to enjoy and live their lives for who they are. Because everyone has that right and should be free to pursue such a goal however they choose, so long as they're not hurting anyone else in the process.

Call *The Myth of Aging* a prescription for that.

After graduating from medical school, I wasn't actually planning on becoming a psychiatrist. I was on track to pursue a career in pediatric medicine, until I learned that a world-famous analyst in Los Angeles had a program that accepted only three people a year. I applied because I'd always been curious about psychiatry, and the analyst, Franz Alexander, had been a disciple of Sigmund Freud. He specialized in psychosomatic psychiatry and psychoanalysis, and I am the last person alive he personally trained. Interestingly, I'd already learned in my internship at Los Angeles County Hospital that a lot of the patients I was seeing were suffering from emotional maladies rooted in problems with their physical health. Working with Franz Alexander reinforced that conclusion and led me to devote my career to not only the patient's mental health but also their physical well-being, because the two are intrinsically tied together.

Eventually, I became a Distinguished Life Fellow of the American Psychiatric Association. I'm also past president of the Southern California Psychoanalytic Institute, where I served as its training and supervising psychoanalyst. I'm a member of the attending staff and teaching faculty of the Cedars-Sinai Medical Center (Emeritus) in Los Angeles and was clinical chief of psychiatry and a member of the Medical Executive Committee of the medical center from 2016 to 2018, and I've published multiple professional papers.

But enough about me. This book is about how I can put my years of experience to work helping you. I don't have a waiting room big enough to accommodate all of you, but this is the next best thing, and I hope you find it helpful.

# PROLOGUE

I did not choose the title *The Myth of Aging* because aging itself is a myth; it quite obviously isn't. The myth lies in how we age from decade to decade, through the milestones of our lives, however we define them for ourselves. No stage of our lives comes without obstacles, setbacks, and challenges, and this book will offer some prescriptions to help you negotiate them so they don't trip you up.

My approach to treating my patients has always offered a holistic approach. In order to help a patient become mentally healthy and aware, I have to be in touch with their physical well-being, in addition to better understanding their emotional life. In other words, if a person is facing mental challenges, then it becomes my responsibility to not only help that person come to grips with the adverse effects physical issues are having on their mental health but also help build a desire and strategy to do something about it. I can't treat the mind without treating the body, because a person's emotional well-being depends on the mind and body being in sync. I have to treat a person in totality.

Don't look at this as a self-help book, though, because it's not. *The Myth of Aging* isn't about instructing you on how to do this or how to do that. Instead, it presents an all-encompassing guide to living the best life you possibly can, both mentally and physically.

In that regard, look at this book as a testament to that symbiosis, an encyclopedia for preserving physical, as well as emotional and mental, health. All forty-three topics contained in the ensuing seven sections may not be of interest to you. But if there's something you need, now you know where you can find it.

Let's start with ten **Do I** questions. Answer each question mentally with a yes or a no.

- Do I wake up in the morning feeling poorly physically or emotionally?
- Do I eat poorly?
- Do I sleep poorly?
- Do I wish my relationships were more fulfilling?
- Do I wish I was happier?
- Do I want to be a better person?
- Do I want to change places with someone else?
- Do I have little to look forward to?
- Do I wish I could do things over again?
- Do I have a lot of regrets?

If you answered yes to two or more of those **Do I** questions, then this book will help you. And if you didn't, then maybe it will help someone you know, perhaps even love. So turn the page and let's begin our session.

# PART ONE

# PHYSICAL AND MENTAL FITNESS

*To keep the body in good health is a duty...otherwise we shall not be able to keep the mind strong and clear.*

—BUDDHA

*I had a patient who came to see me in the wake of suffering a heart attack at the age of sixty-five. Understandably, he was scared and depressed that life as he knew it was over. Even more notably, in facing his own mortality he kept looking away. He was convinced his death was imminent, and there was nothing he could do to prevent it. Most notably, the state of his physical health had led to a steep decline in his mental health as well.*

*I saw him briefly for psychotherapy sessions centered on dying and recovery. The focus of that therapy was to show him his health was very much within his control, that there were steps he could take to recover physically.*

*"What have you been doing for rehab?" I asked him.*

*"Nothing. I tried, but it didn't work so I quit."*

*"What do you mean it didn't work?"*

*"I could only pedal a stationary bike for a few minutes before losing my breath. I thought I was having another heart attack, so I got scared and stopped going."*

*It turned out he was a patient at the hospital I'm affiliated with. I recommended he try their cardiac rehabilitation program and made a contact for him there with someone I knew in that department.*

*"I don't want to see you again until you see him first," I told the patient.*

*He came back the following week, looking and sounding like a different man.*

*"I did five minutes on the bike!" he said, beaming.*

*Two weeks later he was at ten minutes, and a week after that he managed almost twenty. Those might have been small victories, but they were victories all the same, enough for the patient to begin to lose his fear of death, and the remainder of my work with him focused on what additional steps he needed to take in his life to avoid another heart attack caused by the stress that had been consuming him.*

*Getting him to feel better physically allowed me to drill deeper to the source of his stress and anxiety. And once we had dealt with that, he was mentally fit as well. He never came to see me again, but he checks in occasionally to let me know both his physical and mental health are still strong.*

# FINDING YOUR PLACE IN THE WORLD

Finding your place in the world isn't something that only happens to someone on the first leg of life's journey. It's a recurring stop, because as our life changes, that place evolves.

The principles remain the same no matter the stage of life when it occurs. In a time when people are living longer and longer, you may find yourself staking out areas that reflect your sensibility and priorities. The common denominator that runs between them can be described in two words: *purpose* and *belonging*.

Ask yourself, "What excites me to get out of bed in the morning, and what provides comfort, security, and contentment?" Finding your place in the world starts with looking at your life as a zigzagging path across a map. You don't always end up where you expected, and your route constantly changes as your needs and demands change. When patients describe the sense of finding their destination, they inevitably talk about the community of people around them and the inspiration they take from that group. Some discover a new vision for life and a keen sense of self-awareness.

I don't want to provide the false impression that finding your place in the world is easy, though, because it's not. Think of this approach: When your dreams match up with your passion, by pursuing the former, you find the latter. It might not be along the original route you began or in your expected time frame, but there are things you can't map out or set to a clock.

While the steps to find their place in the world vary for everyone, there are a few that act as reliable guideposts along the way.

## PRESCRIPTIONS FOR FINDING YOUR PLACE IN THE WORLD

- **Know who you are:** This is your path, not someone else's. While you can emulate or hold another person in high regard, don't expect the road they took will get you to the same place they reached, any more than you should anticipate reaping the same rewards. Everyone's journey is distinct. If you are constantly comparing yourself to others who've achieved the goals you desire, you may never get where you want to go.
- **Belonging:** Sometimes you don't know who you are until you discover where you belong, as opposed to the opposite. Being a part of something bigger helps set your priorities and define yourself based on them.
- **Your legacy:** Many want to define finding their place in the world as leaving some part of it in better shape than how they found it. It's not just about how you

define yourself but also how others follow your example. Be someone who makes others want to walk in your footsteps and maintain the standards you have set.

- **Being present:** Finding your place in the world encourages you to see life from a different perspective, from the inside looking out rather than the outside looking in. You're in the game instead of merely watching it and changing the score instead of simply following the scoreboard.
- **Stay in motion:** Don't settle for something your heart tells you isn't exactly what you want. Keep moving until you find it. There may be stops along the way, but if you remain where you are because you can't see what's waiting for you over the next ridge, you risk stagnating and may never achieve the happiness that inspires you to grow.
- **Community:** Seek out a community of people who make you want to improve. Mediocrity is not a prescription for optimum mental and emotional health. You've found your place in the world when you surround yourself with others who inspire you to stretch high enough to grasp something you thought was out of your reach.
- **Expand your vision:** The more experiences and the more things you try without fear of failure, the more likely you will find the one that best makes you feel whole. One of the greatest gifts in life at any age is being able to surprise yourself, because that means you haven't stopped growing. And if you keep growing, your place in the world evolves.

- **Familiarity:** I'm not sure where the old saying "familiarity breeds contempt" originated, because in my experience, it breeds comfort and consolation. We are naturally attracted to things in our lives that feel familiar, even when we can't explain why. It just feels like you're meant to be in a specific place or doing a particular thing.
- **Shed your leash:** Avoid the negativity of people who hold you back. Otherwise, you risk becoming a prisoner of someone else's vision. These individuals fear you'll surpass them on whatever road you find yourselves on together. When someone feels they can't succeed unless you fail, that they can't progress unless you recede or stand still, get off that road and find your own.
- **Reach out:** The more you reach out, the more others will reach back. It's not just what you do that helps your mental health but also with whom you do it—maybe even more so, in fact. You're not just seeking a community but building one to help you find your place in the world.

# COPING WITH LONELINESS

Loneliness in society today is pervasive, and its effects on the mind and body aren't restricted by age. Loneliness and its cousin, social isolation, are an equal-opportunity affliction.

According to a recent report issued by the US Department of Health and Human Services, as many as half of all Americans reported regularly experiencing loneliness. For younger people, that number climbs to more than 60 percent. With older people, loneliness tends to be more common among women than men, because men have more opportunities to find someone new than women do. According to that report, "Loneliness and social isolation increase the risk for premature death by 26% and 29% respectively."[1]

I've heard some version of the following from patients for my entire career:

> *I used to have so many friends when I was young, and I had so much fun with them. But the older I get, the less friends and fun I have. I'm not as happy as I used to be because I feel lonely, want to*

> *be like I used to be, and don't know what to do. I don't have the people in my life anymore who make me happy, and I do too much alone....*

What's the prescription for someone dealing with that?

First, I'd want to find out more about what the patient means about being lonely. Is it that they're feeling isolated? Are they depressed and cannot reach out to others? Loneliness is nothing more than a general term; it presents differently in everyone who experiences it.

I had a patient recently, a seventy-year-old man, who came to me because he was feeling lonely and upset, unsettled by the current track his life was on.

"What's your health like?" I asked him.

"Well, I've had two heart attacks, and I have four stents. I really can't get around the way I used to."

This patient had every right to feel depressed and anxious, and I knew I could help him. But will he be as happy as he was when he was forty and in perfect health? No, that's an unrealistic expectation, and I explained to him that happiness means different things at different ages. The fact that he's lost a measure of his health is upsetting, but he should be grateful for the fact that he's walking around and still able to enjoy so many things, even though the list of them is more limited than it used to be. Patients like this man struggling to deal with loneliness need to focus on what they can do and not dwell on what they can't.

With that patient—and anyone reading this book who's dealing with loneliness of any kind—the key is to figure out what they can do to become more engaged and involved in activities that will present opportunities to relieve the sense of isolation roiling them. Start at the root of the problem. Are you lonely because of the loss of a loved one? Are you lonely because some level of physical decline keeps you from doing the things you used to enjoy?

In an article titled "Solitary Man" for KFF Health News, Judith Graham places some of the blame, for men anyway, on "the decline of civic institutions where men used to congregate—think of the Elks or the Shriners—and older men's reduced ability to participate in athletic activities, and the result is a lack of stimulation and the loss of a sense of belonging. Of all age groups in the United States, men over 75 have the highest suicide rate, by far."[2]

You can't play tennis anymore, but what about pickleball? You can't play golf anymore, but what about watching a PGA tournament with the same group you used to share your weekends with on the links? The key to avoiding, or dealing with, loneliness is not to fixate on what you can't fix but to find new ways to enjoy yourself. Look forward instead of back, because the people you're missing aren't returning. Try something new, and you'll meet people with the same experience, regardless of age.

If you come to me and tell me all the negative things going on in your life, I'll say to you, "Okay, I get it, but now tell me how we can fix this and make you grateful for all the positive things you have in life." There is no point in dwelling on negativity. Focus on what you have instead of what you don't. It comes down to finding a different way of approaching how to live life better by focusing on the positive, not the negative.

But you don't need me to help you—you can do it yourself, and here are some of the ways.

## PRESCRIPTIONS FOR COPING WITH LONELINESS

- **Common interests:** One strategy is to seek others with whom you already share interests. Do you like to play chess, read, watch movies and sporting events, or study history? You can find other like-minded individuals on Facebook group pages, at Meetup.com, or within local hobby groups. So many who love reading these days, for example, belong to book clubs that meet monthly. Situations like that provide opportunities to interact with people you can build a connection with over a common interest. It could just as easily be a pickup basketball group or a fan page devoted to your favorite music artists. These people wouldn't be there if they didn't already share something in common with you.
- **Volunteer:** This too should be something you already have an interest in. If you're passionate about the environment, sign up to clear brush to prevent more trees from being lost to fires. Or maybe sign up to teach some kind of hobby you've mastered in a community setting. Consider offering yourself as a guest speaker at a local school to talk about some particular interest or experience that would be appropriate for an educational setting. The sky is pretty much the limit here.
- **Become a joiner:** There are clubs and classes of interest you can sign up for that will create a sense of community for you outside of the virtual world. The key here once more is that you will be in a room of people with whom you have something in common. The sense

of community you get from that may be enough on its own, or you may click with someone in the group, which develops into a friendship beyond the gathering space.

- **Make the call:** Don't wait for someone you'd like to connect with to call you. Take the initiative and make the call yourself. With patients whose depression or anxiety is rooted in loneliness, my prescription for them, instead of antidepressant medications, is to make a minimum of three calls per week, or before our next session. I want them, and you, to take the initiative to engage with others.
- **Social media:** Speaking of clicking, patients of all ages tell me about meeting someone online. They may have lost their partner to death or divorce and had no idea how to meet someone until a friend or acquaintance recommended a matchmaking site to them. People are not always honest in that context, and you must be alert for romance scams, but I am amazed at how many relationships that begin in that manner endure.[3]
- **Pets:** My wife and I were in Miami Beach recently, dining at this excellent Italian restaurant. A woman who had a small dog tucked into a stroller alongside her was sitting alone a few tables over. She was having lunch and a glass of wine, and she talked to the dog through much of her meal as if it were a person. My point in relating this experience was that the woman may have been managing her loneliness with the company of a pet. And while I'm not advocating for you to take your pet out to dinner with you, having a dog, cat, or any animal can be a great prescription to ward

off loneliness. Be warned, though: Pets come with great responsibility, but it's more than justified if they provide you with comfort and solace you might otherwise go without.

# IS PSYCHOTHERAPY FOR YOU?

I wrote this book as a mind, body, and spirit repair manual. Some people, though, may need more than what its pages offer or prefer trying psychotherapy with a trained therapist.

I always recommend looking elsewhere to find the mental stability you feel you're missing. That could be through yoga, Pilates, or meditation and general mindfulness, because these days you may not find what you're looking for on the proverbial psychiatrist's couch. Unfortunately, too many practitioners care about getting you through their door and keeping you there instead of caring about whether you're a good candidate for psychotherapy. They need every patient they can get and keep them as long as possible to pay their overhead and insurance, among other expenses. Many are not prone to advising that a different approach might suit you better.

How should you take the first step to seek a psychologist, psychiatrist, or counselor if you feel the need exists?

For years I've been telling new patients on their first visit, let's see if psychotherapy is right for you, but let's limit it to ten sessions and see if we can make any breakthroughs within that frame. If we haven't, then you know either I'm not the right therapist for you or psychotherapy in general isn't right for your needs.

For it to work, you must feel connected to your therapist. And if you don't feel connected, then chances are you need to find another. Don't make the mistake of believing that the process is supposed to be uncomfortable; it's not. In that respect, shopping for the right therapist who fits your needs and with whom you feel an almost immediate connection is essential. I can often tell in the first ten minutes of a session with a new patient whether I'm the right fit for them, and more times than I can count, the patient had the same feeling but was reluctant to voice it. "Listen," I tell those for whom the fit is wrong, "I don't think you feel connected to me. It's not as if you're wrong or I'm wrong; it's just the way it goes. I have a couple of other therapists to refer you to, and I urge you to shop around and see if there's someone who can fill your needs better than I can."

How do you choose a therapist and know if you've made the right choice?

My advice is to shop around. Many people rely on online reviews to steer them in the right direction, but I've never heard of anyone choosing a therapist that way. Trust your instincts, and if you're not feeling good about the relationship after the first few sessions, move on and try someone else.

How, though, do you know when you should consider seeing someone like me? Here's a list of behavioral triggers that answer the question, especially if you're exhibiting several. Let's call this the **Do you have** list, and if you check two or more, you should consider seeing a mental health professional. So *do you have…*

- Persistent anxiety, sadness, or worry
- A desire to explore what makes you tick
- Panic attacks that seem to get worse
- Thoughts of suicide
- A problem with drugs or alcohol
- An inability to consistently control your emotions
- Inexplicable episodes of anger or rage
- Excessive or irrational fears of things outside your control
- Prolonged grief
- Inability to cope with trauma
- Mood swings that are troubling

In the event you decide to try psychotherapy, here are some of the results you should be looking for.

## PRESCRIPTIONS FOR SUCCESSFUL PSYCHOTHERAPY

- **Chemistry:** Finding the right therapist can be a lot like finding the right partner—you'll know it when you feel it. If you want to see results, you need to have confidence that this is the person who can get you there. For some people, ask yourself if the therapist is someone you'd like to have a drink or a meal with. For others, ask yourself if this is someone who reminds you of a teacher or mentor who made a previous positive impact on your life. Referrals can be effective, but the perfect therapist is the one who is perfect for you.
- **Expectations:** The clearer your goals are when you begin psychotherapy, the more likely you are to realize them. Expressing those expectations to your therapist

will help them develop a program that maximizes the opportunities for success.

- **Don't play doctor:** When the first thing a patient says to me is, "I need to be put on an antidepressant," I point them to the door. If you've predetermined that medication is all that's going to help you, then you're far less likely to be looking for psychotherapy. I don't believe in masking the symptoms. I believe the best results are achieved by addressing the problem itself. I also believe there are times when medication is warranted, and if I'm uncomfortable prescribing it, I will refer the patient to someone who is more willing to do so.
- **Communication:** Someone like me can help you only if you are honest and up-front about why you came in. Sometimes, even frequently, I see patients who don't know why they're not feeling as well as they want to. That's why the aforementioned chemistry between patient and therapist is so vital, because it allows the proper diagnosis to emerge over the initial sessions. But be warned: Just because you communicate what you feel is your problem doesn't mean you've properly identified it.
- **Commitment:** Psychotherapy is not something you can sample here and there. If you want it to be effective, you need to commit yourself to the effort and stick with it in the event you don't see the results you're looking for overnight. And, after a few sessions, try a different therapist if the chemistry between the two of you isn't there. Over the years, a good portion of my patients had tried someone else before they came to me.

- **Have a plan:** After an initial session or two, work with your therapist to lay out the parameters of what your goals are and what you want to achieve from therapy. You go to a physical therapist to get a prescribed plan to help restore the function of a specific part of your body. You go to a psychotherapist to get a comparable plan to help address a specific problem, or problems, with your mind.
- **Medication:** Just because I avoid prescribing drugs like antidepressants doesn't mean they're not right for some patients. In fact, there are many drugs on the market with proven track records of helping patients. The key for your therapist is to determine if drug therapy is right for you and, if so, which drug will provide the best results. I'm also very interested in the progress being made with the use of drugs such as ketamine and psilocybin in treating depression especially.
- **Alternative therapies:** If you're suffering from depression, your therapist may recommend, or you may want to ask them about, newer approaches to treatment like TMS, or transcranial magnetic stimulation, which works by using magnetic waves or pulses to stimulate the brain's nerve cells. One note of caution: Therapies like TMS and others should not be used as a first line of defense but rather for those patients who haven't responded to more traditional therapies.

# DEALING WITH CHANGE

Imagine if change could happen instantly—if we could wake up one day and simply decide, "Today, I'll start eating healthier," and then follow through effortlessly, or say, "I'm going to quit smoking," and never touch a cigarette again.

But we know that change doesn't work that way. It is not a single decision or one-time act. Change is a gradual process. The more we understand this journey, the more we can show empathy, offer support, and practice compassion for ourselves and others striving to make meaningful changes.

Change can be good and positive. It's a part of life as we grow and evolve, neither of which ever stops. Embracing change might just be the best recipe to prevent the worst effects of aging, because nothing is more emotionally and psychologically destructive than stubbornly clinging to the status quo, even when it's not working anymore.

You need to be capable of changing as I was back when I was fifty-six years old. At that point, I knew I needed to alter my life significantly. Even though I was uncomfortable with those changes initially, they proved to be beneficial to the point where I'm not sure I'd be writing this book to help you today otherwise.

Upheaval, on the other hand, is not good. Upheaval refers to everything going upside down in your life, and that's when you may need some help. It's essential to be able to distinguish between change and upheaval. Change is something a person decides to do. It's consciously determined, as opposed to being brought on by random factors outside your control or the actions of others.

An example would be a man or woman who likes their life but finds themselves in a marriage or relationship that they no longer find fulfilling. So they decide to work on their marriage or relationship, to change something. If that doesn't work, they may make a more significant change by dissolving the marriage.

In opposition to that scenario, one spouse may catch the other having a long-time affair or the other spouse may come clean about it. A marriage where they were likely happy for a long time ends tumultuously in contention and strife. That's upheaval, which is very hard to embrace or accept. Change might also be downsizing to a smaller home after the kids are gone and a couple's lifestyle has evolved. Upheaval would be the house burning down with all the same couple's worldly possessions lost forever.

Upheaval is sad, depressing, and potentially annihilating. This is when you may need to seek the help of a trained psychotherapist who understands what you're going through. Thanks to events beyond your control, you may have lost yourself. You're wandering and need some direction. In that case, you'd turn to a therapist or counselor to help you get back on the right track.

It's important to distinguish between change you can affect and change forced on you by sickness, an accident, death, or some combination, like the tragic fires in Los Angeles in early 2025. That kind of catastrophe tests our mettle most severely, and there is no straightforward prescription to deal with it. Sometimes being strong for others is the most positive approach you can take. People are able to manage that, but they may crumble when left to face their grief and sense of loss alone. When a son, daughter, close friend, or spouse is dealing with a serious illness, your salvation can be remaining strong for them, casting yourself as the rock they need. Even if all you can do is visit them every day and do your best to keep their spirits high enough, that's a great thing for your loved one and a recipe for preserving your mental and emotional health.

I'd also strongly advise you not to lose yourself helping someone else or responding to an upheaval thrust upon you. That's when you need to keep to your exercise routine as much as possible. And if you don't have one, now might be the perfect time to start one to create a much-needed mental distraction. To be there for your loved ones, you must also be there for yourself. If your health—emotionally, mentally, and physically—deteriorates, you lose the ability to do what you've committed yourself to doing. It's not a question of being selfish so much as being smart.

Positive change can also be disquieting and, for some people, even destructive. Too often, those who experience a financial windfall that changes their life are ill-equipped to handle it. They end up undoing the good that has happened. That's a perfect time for the mental reset that could include therapy to ensure you stay on track, even if it's down another road. Over the years, I've seen too many people who've let money change who they are. They come to me and say something like, "I was happier before." I ask them why, what they feel they're missing now, and how they can get it back without sacrificing any gains. Self-realization can go a long way in addressing this, though this scenario may be one where therapy is warranted.

## PRESCRIPTIONS FOR DEALING WITH CHANGE

- **Acceptance:** Before you can positively respond to change, you first have to accept it. The absolute worst way to deal with change is to remain in denial about it or believe things will return to how they were. That is impossible, and the best remedy for it is to focus forward, not back.
- **Adjust and adapt:** Dancers talk about the need to be light on their feet to pull off the most challenging of moves. So, too, we must be light on our feet when facing a change we didn't ask for but is now a part of our lives. The more flexible and permeable you are, the better you can handle even the most challenging aspects of change.
- **Think positive:** You are the same person you were before the change happened. Focus on other times in your life when you were able to make lemonade out of lemons to build the confidence you can do it again or more successfully than the last time.
- **Rely on your rocks:** Focus on the parts of your life that offer stability and you can cling to even when change strips away one of those rocks. Life isn't a sprint, it's a

marathon, and if you have assembled enough anchors along the way, you'll be able to cope when one breaks free.

- **Give it time:** Time can't heal everything, but it can make even the most drastic change more tolerable with its passing.
- **Don't overreact:** Outside of a few of the most drastic changes we may face, things are often not nearly as bad as they initially seem. Let things sink in and focus your energies on what can be gained instead of what change has taken from you. Keep things in their proper perspective, and have a sensible conversation with yourself about what will be different and how you can best cope with that.

# THE IMPORTANCE OF EXERCISE

The term "self-esteem" gets thrown around in psychiatric circles and beyond. But it's extremely relevant in terms of exercise.

Seeing yourself as physically fit, or even somewhat physically fit, will make you feel a lot better about yourself as opposed to not liking what you see when you look in the mirror. This goes to the heart of the holistic mind-body concept that has defined my practice for over half a century.

And yet a 2023 report by the Centers for Disease Control and Prevention (CDC) determined that only 28 percent of Americans over eighteen exercise regularly at sufficient levels.[4] That means nearly three-quarters of the country's population may not like what looks back at them from the mirror, if they ever bother looking at all, a recipe for poor mental health as well as physical. The Department of Health and Human Services recommends that adults should spend no less than 150 minutes per week doing aerobic exercises at a moderate intensity and spend at least two days a week doing resistance training and muscle-strengthening activities like lifting weights.[5]

A deeper dive into the demographics is striking. The statistics above are disheartening enough, even before considering that the CDC estimates that less than one-quarter of all children between six and seventeen years old exercise at least sixty minutes daily.[6] Blame cell phones, video games, and social media if you want, but the priorities of kids, adults, and seniors need to change. CDC stands for Centers for Disease Control and *Prevention*, and there is no better way to prevent mental illness and preserve cognitive health than by establishing a regular exercise routine. That will potentially bring up the numbers I just quoted.

Oftentimes, with adults as young as thirty, exercise can be a matter of managing expectations. I can't tell you how often I've asked a patient suffering from depression what they do for exercise. Usually, the answer I get is something along the lines of, "Well, not much anymore, because I can't do what I used to do. It hurts too much, and I keep getting injured." In that regard, establishing the kind of exercise routine vital for preserving mental health is a matter of managing expectations.

- If you can't play racquetball anymore, try pickleball.
- If you can't run, walk.
- If you can't play baseball, join a softball league.
- If swimming bothers your shoulders, alternate between swimming laps or walking them.

Remember to take it easy at first and stretch, when recommitting yourself to an exercise regimen. And don't be afraid to try something new. Taking on a new activity is not only great for the body but also for the mind.

We have an excellent gym in the apartment building where my wife and I live. Sometimes, I'm not even the oldest one working out, even though many people I see on weight machines can't lift their own weight. But that doesn't matter, because studies increasingly show the value of resistance training for older adults, even among those who've never lifted weights before. Some residents of my gym prefer dumbbells, resistance bands, or cardio machines. Most opt for a steady mix, often varying their routine over multiple days of the week. The common denominator between all of them is they always leave the gym with a smile on their face. Happy, fulfilled, and feeling good about themselves. There's simply no better recipe for mental health than that. You don't have to do a lot or train excessively hard. You must know your limits and come to grips with the fact that exercise is not a one-size-fits-all activity. You need to find what works for you and what you enjoy enough to return.

One unfortunate trend recently noted by *The New York Times* is that women exercise at lower rates, 33 to 43 percent, than men.[7] That's interesting because, on average, women live six years more than men. Given that, the adage "it's not the years in your life but the life in your years" could never be more accurate. Living a long life without sufficient exercise and remaining sedentary too much is likely to affect your quality of life profoundly. You won't feel good mentally if you don't feel good physically. I don't usually speak in absolutes, but in this case it's accurate.

## PRESCRIPTIONS FOR MAKING EXERCISE A PART OF YOUR LIFE

- **Stress relief:** I don't know of anything better to relieve the daily and even greater stressors that can disrupt our lives. No problem seems as big after a workout as it did before.

- **Mood management:** Exercising makes you feel better about pretty much everything. It takes your mind off whatever was plaguing you when you started your workout. The problem will still be there when you finish, but you'll look at it with a different and more positive, or at least objective, perspective.
- **Taking a mental vacation:** Concentrating on physical exertion to manage a specific task turns the focus of your mind outward from inward. You're counting reps in the weight room, miles on the street, or rowing strokes instead of adding up all your problems.
- **Better sleep:** Exercise boosts almost everything to the point where you're more tired and thus ready to slip off to sleep when the time comes.
- **Enhanced self-esteem:** Nothing makes you feel better than practicing your exercise routine with diligence and consistency. Even when the weather's lousy or you're dead tired, pushing yourself to work out is a priority that makes others seem less important by comparison.
- **Confidence:** You don't have to be a bodybuilder, marathon runner, or competitive racquet sports player to build confidence in yourself; the same goal can be achieved merely by practicing the act itself. Having the confidence to compete, win or lose, leaves us more confident about everything we do.

# YOUR MEAL TICKET TO HEALTHY EATING

Nothing is more important than diet when maintaining your mental and physical health. And, unfortunately, the diets boasted by too many of us are lacking, often woefully so. We overeat what we shouldn't and don't eat enough of what we should.

"There is growing recognition of the role of nutrition in mental health," Marta Mudd wrote in *Psychiatric News* in January 2025. "Poor dietary habits are now understood as modifiable risk factors for mental health. Further, research suggests that individuals with psychiatric illness are more likely to have poor dietary patterns, disordered eating behaviors, and nutritional deficiency, contributing to both physical and mental health comorbidities. Therefore, there is an urgent need to integrate lifestyle interventions such as nutrition management in treating psychiatric illness."[8]

Many consider the rising rates of obesity in America, for example, to be a public health crisis. The statistics are devastating. The CDC estimates the prevalence of obesity to be between

40 and 45 percent of the population, a staggering figure, to say the least.[9] But that's not even the worst news. The National Institutes of Health has reported that between 20 and 60 percent of persons suffering from obesity are also afflicted with some form of psychiatric illness or impairment. Those include depression, eating disorders, anxiety, and substance abuse.[10]

That makes no mention of what being overweight does to a person's quality of life. People who are overweight tend to be fearful of being shamed or stigmatized, so they are less likely to seek social outlets. I haven't seen any studies about this, but my guess is those who are overweight spend far more time alone and/or in their homes, which can be highly detrimental to their mental health as well.

Healthy body, healthy mind. I can't say it enough.

A lousy diet becomes a self-fulfilling prophecy, setting off a spiral where you can develop many other health issues. Bad diets, for instance, explain the epidemic of type 2 diabetes in this country. In that regard, there is hope in the form of the drug semaglutide, prescribed to overweight patients under the trade names Ozempic and Wegovy. The problem is these drugs haven't been around long enough to have a clear notion of their long-term side effects. They also provide the wrong impression that excellent health is only a pill or an injection away, which is the antithesis of the holistic approach to mental fitness I use in my practice. These drugs, in my mind, are the physiological equivalent of antidepressants for those who come to me because they're depressed. They can produce excellent results for those who need them the most, but they should be regarded as a last resort instead of a first.

Over my career, when I've taken on a new patient, I make it a point to get a detailed medical history because I want to understand how their mind and body operate in tandem. And that includes their eating habits.

Marta Mudd puts it well in her *Psychiatric News* piece: "Growing evidence indicates that nutritional interventions should play a central role in psychiatric care. This emerging body of research highlights the importance of improving diet quality, adopting specific dietary patterns, and incorporating supplements when appropriate to support mental health outcomes. By incorporating nutrition management into routine care using existing resources, psychiatrists can empower patients to take charge of both their mental and physical health."[11]

## PRESCRIPTIONS FOR HEALTHY EATING

- **Planning and preparation:** The best way to maintain a healthy diet is not to wait until the last minute to plan your meals. Whether you are cooking, ordering in, or purchasing prepared meals, have a notion, at the very least, of what you're going to eat for dinner so you can balance your other food selections for the day accordingly.
- **Eat more fruits and vegetables:** First off, don't be discouraged if you're not meeting someone else's benchmarks. That's why I'm not even listing how many portions are recommended by what sources. A good rule of thumb is to make a habit of snacking on fruit instead of candy, chips, or other processed foods. As for the amount of fruits and vegetables, do the best you can but don't stress if that occasionally turns out to

fall a bit short. And don't be afraid to give nutritional supplements a try to see if they're the right fit for you.

- **Experiment with diets:** There are a ton of new approaches to dietary change out there to try if you want. Among the readily available options are the Mediterranean diet, the DASH diet (Dietary Approaches to Stop Hypertension), the MIND diet (Mediterranean-DASH Intervention for Neurodegenerative Delay), as well as the ketogenic diet.[12] There are numerous others, the most important factor being to settle on one you can stick with.
- **Consult with a nutritionist:** Sometimes the advice and wisdom of a trained professional can provide both information and motivation for eating healthier. A trained nutritionist can also help you sort through the various options out there and help you find the one that's best for you.
- **Be realistic:** Know who you are. For some, portion control might be the best approach. For others, a more radical approach might work, like it does for the great Bruce Springsteen, who eats only one meal a day. I have a patient who's found great success in steadily losing weight by committing to a diet in which he finishes dinner by 4:00 p.m. every day to allow optimum time between then and the following day's breakfast. Just don't assume what works for someone else is going to work for you in the long term.
- **Moderation:** Yes, you should eat more fish, but that doesn't mean you have to give up red meat entirely. Cutting back on meat from twice a week to once, or even three times a week to twice, means you're

committed to improving, and that makes for a great start. The pace at which you change your diet to adopt a healthier lifestyle does not require you to make radical changes that are less likely to last. I've found a far better approach is to build your diet around what you love eating, but potentially less often and as part of a more balanced diet.

- **Cut back on sugar and fats:** Definitely cut back, but patients I've had who try to quit sugar and fats cold turkey seldom maintain their commitment. Remember that every little bit you do can add up to a lot.
- **Do your research:** New recommendations and advice for building better health with what you put in your body are coming all the time, so keep your mind open to trying new things and even taking a fresh look at something old. "What is a societally condoned dietary constituent that helps prevent liver disease, makes you alert, and does not need to break the bank?" asks Jasmohan S. Bajaj, a hepatologist and professor at Virginia Commonwealth University. "Coffee! The cheapest brewed coffee with the lowest number of additives helps the brain, liver, and microbiota."[13]

# MINDFULNESS

As a psychiatrist who has long resisted prescribing antidepressant and antianxiety medication for my patients, I'm always looking for drug-free therapies that can achieve comparable results. One of those therapies getting a lot of attention these days is something called "mindfulness."

Mindfulness is a form of meditation anyone can practice, designed to help you focus on the present moment. That makes perfect sense to me, given that so much of the stress and anxiety I've long seen in my patients is based on regret over the past and worry over the future. By focusing on the present, you learn to live in and appreciate the now, instead of what's been and what's coming. The fact that we can't do anything about what's been and really don't know what's coming doesn't stop us from stressing out over both.

"It's the nature of the mind to think, analyze, and figure things out," Crystal Hoshaw wrote for the website Healthline in March 2022. "That's its job. That means that left to its own devices, the mind will constantly seek out new stimuli, new things to think about, and new ways to check out from reality. Mindfulness practice is a way to gently retrain the mind to settle into the present moment. It's kind of like becoming a parent to your mind rather than letting it control you. In the end, the mind is simply a willful toddler. By practicing mindfulness over and over with patience and compassion for yourself, you can teach the mind to be still."[14]

According to the American Psychological Association, "Mindfulness is awareness of one's internal states and surroundings. Mindfulness can help people avoid destructive or automatic habits and responses by learning to observe their thoughts, emotions, and other present-moment experiences without judging or reacting to them. Mindfulness is used in several therapeutic interventions, including mindfulness-based cognitive behavior therapy, mindfulness-based stress reduction, and mindfulness meditation."[15]

But does it actually work?

Recent studies, including one conducted at Georgetown University Medical Center (as published in *JAMA Psychiatry*), have found that mindfulness can be as or more effective than prescription medications in treating anxiety and depression.[16]

"Although the new study was the first clinical trial to directly compare medication and mindfulness as treatments for anxiety disorders," Kaitlin Sullivan wrote in *Health* in a November 2022 article, "mounting research on the topic for the past decade has suggested mindfulness and meditation can help rework a person's relationship with their anxiety for the better. A study published last year in the journal *PLOS One* included 190 medical professionals who work in emergency rooms. The researchers found that those who practiced mindfulness were less likely to experience both anxiety and depression. Additionally, a review in *Current Psychology*, also published last year, included 11 studies on mindfulness and anxiety in an attempt to determine how the practice works to reduce symptoms."[17]

So that's what mindfulness can accomplish, but how can you practice it?

## PRESCRIPTIONS FOR PRACTICING MINDFULNESS

- **Breathing:** Like all forms of meditation, mindfulness relies heavily on getting to a place in your mind and body where your breathing is smooth and steady. Breathing in this manner stimulates awareness of your inner physical and emotional self. With each breath and beat of your heart, you are retreating further inside yourself, with the physical world becoming less and less important as time seems to freeze in a moment of peace and solitude where you are unburdened.
- **Focus:** This is not the time to fixate on the woes that may be plaguing you. It's the time to view those woes in a larger context that trains your focus away from what you can't control and in full command of what you can. You may hear a bird singing or music playing somewhere nearby, but avoid any outside stimulus of your own making. Put your cell phone in another room, and choose a setting, indoors or out, that already serves as a comfort zone for you. But no distractions!
- **Practice:** As in any new activity, it's going to take some time to become proficient at mindfulness. The best way to improve is to build mindfulness sessions into your schedule, preferably around the same time(s)

every day. You may want to try five minutes at first, then ten, and then fifteen before ultimately settling on the time frame that's best for you. There are a ton of articles online that offer advice from those who've made mindfulness a part of their everyday lives and can help you learn to do the same.

- **Savor:** Mindfulness isn't just an exercise; it can also be a lifestyle. When you're out walking, take time to savor the beauty around you. When you're dining, take time to savor how good your favorite meal or dessert tastes. Enjoy and appreciate experiences you normally take for granted to help reset your priorities and put things in their proper perspective—all told, a great recipe for avoiding depression, stress, and anxiety.
- **Experiment:** You may find that you get better results from practicing mindfulness while you're engaged in some type of physical activity like walking, running, or some form of noncompetitive martial art like tai chi or aikido. You may find practicing mindfulness in a dark room gets you the greatest results. You may find those same results are best achieved on a sandy beach with only the sound of the waves and the wind in your ears. Try different approaches, even a combination of them, to find which gets your emotional state where it needs, and you want it, to be.
- **The Five R's:** In November 2022, City Center Psychotherapy identified the Five R's of mindfulness: Recognize, Relax, Review, Respond, and Return. Full explanations of each can be found at the link in the endnote, but generally the Five R's provide a kind of agenda to keep you grounded and on point when

practicing mindfulness. But don't feel an obligation to stick to that prescribed protocol. You may eventually settle on a methodology of your own that gets you to the same place.[18]

# PART TWO

# RESILIENCE

*Do not judge me by my success, judge me by how many times I fell down and got back up again.*

—NELSON MANDELA

*I saw a young man for several years who was suffering from acute trauma as a result of being abandoned as an infant. The residue of that experience had led to him suffering extreme anxiety, alienation, and the feeling he could never be good enough for himself or anyone else. Lacking the resilience to overcome that trauma, he had trouble committing to school and work and was deeply disturbed by his lack of strong relationships, especially with women.*

*"Why do you think you were abandoned as an infant?" I asked him, early in his psychotherapy.*

*"Because my parents, maybe just my mother, couldn't provide for me."*

*"So it had nothing to do with who you were. It was about who they were."*

*"I guess."*

*And yet the root of the problem was that he blamed himself for being abandoned. I focused his therapy for a time on the things he had accomplished, to show how resilient he could be until the trauma resurfaced. We needed to work on reducing the impact that trauma was having on his life. That meant sessions aimed at boosting his self-esteem and seeking valves he could turn to release the trauma when it returned.*

*"What makes you feel the best about yourself?"*

*"I like working with kids. I've thought about teaching."*

*That figured, given that his own trauma was rooted in his childhood.*

*"I wish I could do for them what you're doing for me," he added, unprompted.*

*Well into his therapy, this patient went back to school and stayed there this time, having found the resilience that ultimately led to him becoming a successful child therapist who is still practicing today.*

# FINANCIAL SETBACKS

If you're concerned about money, you're not alone. People from all backgrounds struggle with financial stress and uncertainty in these challenging times. Whether your worries stem from job loss, rising debt, unexpected expenses, or a combination of issues, financial stress is one of the most common pressures in modern life. Even before the global coronavirus pandemic and its economic consequences, a study by the American Psychological Association (APA) revealed that 72 percent of Americans experienced financial stress at least occasionally.[19] Periodic, inevitable economic downturns only intensify these struggles for many.

Like other overwhelming stressors, financial difficulties can significantly impact your mental and physical well-being, relationships, and overall quality of life. Constant money worries can disrupt sleep, lower self-esteem, and drain energy. They can lead to feelings of anger, shame, or fear, cause tension and arguments with loved ones, and even worsen physical pain, mood swings, and mental health conditions such as depression and anxiety. In some cases, people may turn to unhealthy coping mechanisms like substance abuse or gambling to escape their problems. At its most severe, financial stress can trigger suicidal thoughts or actions. However, no matter how dire your situation may feel, there are healthier ways to cope. By addressing your financial challenges directly, you can reduce stress, regain control of your finances, and improve your overall well-being.[20]

The ramifications of financial setbacks are not limited to a dwindling bank account. They can also eat away at your mental and even physical health. I have had patients dealing with money problems who have experienced insomnia, depression, anxiety, relationship struggles, and social isolation. From a physical standpoint, I've seen patients with migraines, digestive problems, diabetes, high blood pressure, and heart disease. And I've also seen how these problems can be further accentuated by abusing alcohol and drugs. Those experiencing financial issues might have to cancel their gym membership because they can't afford it anymore, and the same holds true for being able to maintain a healthy diet. It costs more to eat well, and many of the patients who've articulated having financial issues have gotten away from eating patterns that help ensure good health.

Financial problems are a prime example of how psychological issues manifest physically, further demonstrating the inexorable link between the mind and the body. Some patients I've seen in this space have experienced financial reversals through no fault of their own. They have been swindled, scammed, or conned the way the Ponzi scheme victims of Bernie Madoff were. Others have made bad investments or experienced financial hardships due to declining health, forcing them to cut back or leave the business altogether. Ironically, too many successful people prioritize money so much that they fail to take care of their physical health and, as a result, lose both simultaneously.

Many of these people weren't living within their financial means to begin with, spending money based on expectations rather than reality. I might say to them, "I understand how important money is to you, but tell me some other things that are also important." And then I try to make them see that so much more they hold dear remains in their grasp. I might advise them to visit a financial counselor to help them figure out how to live with less and how to budget as well as downsize appropriately.

I recommend several strategies for bouncing back from financial calamities or limiting the toll they take. Let's call them the Four A's.

## PRESCRIPTIONS FOR DEALING WITH FINANCIAL HARDSHIP

- **Acceptance:** Like any negatives that befall us in life, acceptance of our current state is necessary before moving on. Living in the present while fixating on the past and whatever wrongs may have transpired will only result in doing continued harm to your mental and physical health. There are no good ways to deal with the lifestyle changes that financial calamity forces on us. Before we can chart a new course to move forward, though, we must stop looking back to make the most of the cards that have been dealt to us.
- **Assessment:** There's a balance sheet in life, and I stress to my patients the importance of highlighting the positive aspects of their lives versus the negative. In the case of a severe financial setback, we must take a figurative assessment and make it literal. What resources do you still have, and how much debt are you carrying? Is taking advantage of the bankruptcy laws an option? What

are your options for new earnings? How much can you downsize while preserving a different quality of life? What is your legal recourse if you've been wronged? Don't be afraid to seek professional advice to help you answer these questions.

- **Action:** This refers to putting the plan derived from your assessment into action. Not everything is guaranteed to go smoothly, so you may need to adjust on the fly. So, too, you need to be up-front with your spouse and children about how this may affect their responsibilities and expectations. By the same token, though, suffering a financial calamity is the time to come together as a family and not splinter apart, which will only further exacerbate the physical and mental toll the experience takes on all involved.
- **Attitude:** It's hard to be optimistic and look at the world through rose-colored glasses when the lenses are cracked. The more you focus on what you still have, as opposed to what you've lost, the stronger you will emerge. And the better your mental, physical, and emotional health is going into a crisis, the more able you will be to emerge positively on the other side. When patients talk to me about the financial issues plaguing them, I'll often ask them about something else entirely, like relationships with their children and friends. I want to get them talking about something positive in their lives that's still there to provide context to what they've lost. Life is about the people you love, not about the stuff you have, and I've had patients who emerge on the other side of a financial calamity with a whole new attitude and reset of their priorities.

# COPING WITH RETIREMENT

Over the years, I've had many patients who've either retired or were on the verge of doing so. Coming from a man still seeing patients after fifty or so years practicing psychiatry, I might offer myself up as an example here.

I'm still working because I love what I do and believe I remain good at it. I think I can continue to make a difference in the lives of those who come to me for help, and in doing so, I find purpose, direction, and meaning. I wake up on work mornings with the tremendous responsibility of having patients trust me with their innermost thoughts to help improve their lives. I wouldn't trade that for anything and can't imagine waking up every morning without such a thing to look forward to.

According to WebMD, in an article titled "The Emotional Shock of Retirement," one in three retirees reported feeling depressed.[21] But there's a prescription to prevent that, which starts with PREPARATION. I capitalized that because I can't stress enough that preparation is vital in planning your post-working life.

There's another P word to stress as well: PURPOSE. Find a sense of purpose. It could be volunteering actively for a cause you've long supported, teaching kids to read, babysitting your grandchildren, or serving on a board at your place of worship. How about supporting a political campaign? Giving back that way not only occupies your time but also fulfills your need to have an impact and continue to make a difference, which is an excellent strategy for preserving your mental and emotional health.

Exploring new hobbies or interests can be another great option. You could try painting, working with stained glass, or taking a class on a subject that has always interested you. In that regard, a key prescription for navigating retirement is establishing a new routine to replace your old one. It might feel good to wake up with nothing to do for a while, but trust me, it won't last.

What's right for me, though, isn't right for everybody, so I'd like to provide a checklist for those contemplating retirement, those who miss their old lives, and those who define themselves so much by their work that they can't let it go, even to the detriment of their mental and physical health.

## PRESCRIPTIONS FOR RETIREMENT

- **Do you love what you do?** Nothing is more important than this when weighing your decision. If you still find your work gratifying and fulfilling, why retire?
- **Are you still good at what you do?** Even if you still enjoy what you're doing, you have to be honest with yourself about the quality and quantity of your work. Ask yourself if you're as productive and efficient as you were five, ten, fifteen, or twenty years ago. Your

productivity is a by-product of your continuing passion for what you do.

- **Are you physically and mentally capable of continuing to do what you do?** Like me, many of us work in professions that are not physically taxing. And working late into life can be the best way to preserve your mental acuity. When it comes to more physically demanding professions, it's a matter of learning to pace yourself and, on your days off, to find activities that relax your body as well as your mind. In other words, give yourself time to recover.
- **What will your life look like if you stop what you're doing?** This is a big one, because how exactly will you occupy your time when you're not working? Do you have hobbies or pursuits you enjoy as much as your work? What will your days look like? There's an old saying that you should never throw out your dirty water until you have clean water to replace it. In that regard, you should not wait until retirement to plan for what your life will look like afterward.
- **How will you spend your time if you stop?** I've had colleagues who've moved into teaching or mentoring. Some have dedicated themselves to volunteering or fulfilling their long-held dreams to travel the world. A few have written books, while others are on the golf course five days a week, or out sailing. There's no right or wrong answer here, but some advice I give my patients is to be excited about how they will spend their day and make sure they find something as fulfilling as their former work to maintain their mental health.

- **What are the financial expectations after retirement?** Some people can't retire, even if they want to, either because they haven't planned their finances properly or have encountered a financial setback. Another thing I ask my patients is if they are sure they can maintain the lifestyle they want without working. It makes no sense to retire to play golf when you can't afford to play anymore.
- **How will you replace the intangibles of what you do?** For many of us, our work environment also serves as the basis for our social life or, at least, much of our social interaction. It may seem great to wake up without having to fight traffic to get to the office. Except it's not just about how you will spend the day that follows but also with whom, so you may need to seek out new opportunities to engage with people socially without the workplace environment to do that for you.

# COPING WITH ILLNESS

There is no more wrenching an experience emotionally than dealing with illness—not just your own, of course, but those close to you. I've had many patients through the years whose happy lives have been derailed by disease, decline, and infirmity. It's even more detrimental to your emotional health when it's a spouse, parent, or child who gets sick, casting you in the role of caregiver.

Of course, this is one of the primary reasons why I've long been stressing a holistic approach to health in my practice. The better you feel physically, the better you will feel mentally. And the better shape you're in, the better equipped you will be to deal with the effects of even a serious illness on yourself or a loved one.

Facing such an illness can introduce uncertainty into many areas of life, which might influence your emotions. A sense of control often brings comfort and allows us to enjoy life, so it's natural to want clarity about the future to help plan. A bad diagnosis, however, can disrupt that feeling of control, leaving you unsettled. Dealing with uncertainty is one of the hardest parts of illness, often manifesting in fear, frustration, and/

or anger. Learning more about your condition and discussing potential outcomes with your health-care team can sometimes ease these feelings.

It's often difficult to determine whether a treatment will be entirely successful or if the illness will be cured. Even after completing treatment, concerns about recurrence can linger, making it challenging to look ahead with confidence and leaving you longing for definitive answers. Unfortunately, knowing if an illness has been completely cured is not always possible, especially with cancer. Health-care professionals may not always provide clear answers, and their uncertainty can be frustrating.

Let's look at what to expect and thus work toward avoiding stress when coping with your own illness or that of someone you love.

## PRESCRIPTIONS FOR COPING WITH ILLNESS

- **Anxiety:** I've heard this called "scan-xiety" for cancer patients and their caregivers. It's natural to be anxious when you don't know what's coming next and every bit of good news is tempered by what we can't see around the next corner. There is no remedy for anxiety, but doing as much as you can that's within your control can relieve it. For example, I've had many patients who've been frightened into losing weight and building an exercise regimen after suffering a heart attack or being diagnosed with a heart condition. It's never too late to take as much control as you can over your body or coax a loved one to do the same.

- **Loneliness:** People who are sick often don't want to burden others; they may not even want anyone but their immediate family to know they're ill. The default setting for so many of us is to bear the pain alone, but that's a prescription for letting the disease defeat you or your loved one. I've often recommended joining a support group for patients who express this to me, both during and after treatment. It's good for a patient's mental health to be among like-minded folks who can share their experiences and potentially offer tips and support. Misery, as they say, loves company, but company helps relieve the misery.
- **Anger:** "Why me?" patients often complain. "What did I do to deserve this?" This is a self-destructive impulse, and I tend to be quite firm with patients who express it to me. The most essential thing in this regard is for the patient or caregiver to train their focus forward. Bemoaning or reliving a car accident isn't going to cause the damage to go away, and the same thing holds true here. Train your focus forward and celebrate every victory, no matter how small or fleeting. Recovering alcoholics are presented with chips or coins at weekly and monthly marks to celebrate their ongoing success. It's the same with illness. I've had patients who've entered cardiac rehabilitation programs after suffering a heart attack, and I encourage them to rejoice in something as simple as riding a stationary bike for ten minutes or walking a half mile on a treadmill. The prescription here is celebrating the little things, even in the face of something big.
- **Sorrow:** I see this mostly in family members thrust into the role of caregivers who don't bother to celebrate the

small victories because they are so few and far between. I don't discourage it, because it's as natural as being in pain after breaking a limb, and it often appears as a kind of pre-grieving process in which the caregiver becomes resigned to the inevitability of what's coming. I strongly encourage them to do everything possible to make whoever they're caring for comfortable and loved. Knowing you did everything you possibly could, exhausted every option, and never gave up won't erase your sorrow. But it will make it easier to accept what's coming, because you have maximized what's in your control to affect. Take advantage of every opportunity and make every moment count. The smallest things can sometimes produce profound effects going forward.

- **Depression:** This might be a case where antidepressant drugs are warranted. But it's also an instance that calls for reaching out beyond yourself for help, whether you're the caregiver or the patient. The holistic nature of my practice has resulted in me seeing a multitude of patients in this space, because caring for a loved one has left them in a depressed state. I stress the importance of being at their best to bear the harsh burden they're charged with. That means prioritizing their health through diet and exercise so the dreaded disease doesn't claim two victims instead of one. Depression among those afflicted, meanwhile, is understandably common. When treating the psychological effects of their illness, I urge them to take stock of their lives to focus on all they've achieved and the legacy they've built. And if they cannot articulate that legacy, I help them find it.

# SPIRITUALITY

That, appropriately enough, brings us to spirituality. Notice I didn't say religion, because spirituality means different things to different people. For some people in a situation that requires resilience, seeking comfort from a priest, rabbi, imam, or minister is exactly what this doctor ordered when a patient is already predisposed to that—I don't think religion is necessarily something you gravitate to only when the need arises.

Some people find their spirituality in the practice of yoga or meditation. Think about the various positions and movements of yoga, all aimed at making you suppler and more physically flexible. Well, the very same practice can stimulate the psychological flexibility that makes you resilient and more capable of dealing with setbacks in your life.

Religion can define your sense of spirituality, such as frequenting services at a synagogue or church regularly. All people benefit from believing in something bigger than themselves that better enables them to define their place in the world.

A 2018 study published by the National Institutes of Health produced findings that confirmed a definitive link between spirituality and being more resilient in life. The study concluded that those who considered themselves spiritual were significantly better equipped to deal with hardship and tragedy than those who weren't, going as far as to call such an attitude "a vital component of their resilience, leading to subjective well-being" and that "spiritual resilience is a tool aiding in how the participants recover from adversity, sustain a sense of well-being, and grow spiritually and developmentally as they age."[22]

I think that the final line is crucial, because I often tell my patients that they're never too old to take on something new, including expanding or enhancing their spiritual beliefs and experiences. Sometimes even, the older one gets the more they gravitate toward something that provides community, support, and reinforcement.

Spirituality can make you more resilient by providing a sense of meaning and purpose in life, offering a framework for coping with challenges, fostering a connection to something larger than yourself, and facilitating positive and proactive activities like prayer, meditation, and reflection, which breed inner strength and a wider perspective. Let's explore some of the ways this happens.

## PRESCRIPTIONS FOR PRACTICING SPIRITUALITY

- **Meaning:** Spirituality can help us make sense of events in life that otherwise confound us. Life tends to be composed of some balance of highs and lows. Being spiritual similarly helps us from getting too high in the good times or too low in the bad. It helps retain, or restore, balance to life, and those who accept it into their lives tend to see things in a bigger picture through a more objective lens.

- **Support:** Spirituality can provide comfort and community outside of family and friends. It encourages us to foster relationships with like-minded people who have gathered toward common pursuits and beliefs. There's a reason why attendance in churches and synagogues rises during times of war, strife, and calamity. Nobody wants to feel alone in challenging times.
- **Inner peace:** Spirituality provides perspective, serving to make us aware of a universe in which many wheels are spinning to lift our focus off the wheel that has ground to a halt beneath us. The serenity prayer includes the line, "Accept the things I cannot change, the courage to change the things I can, and the wisdom to know the difference." That mantra serves as an abstract definition of resilience.
- **Coping:** Similarly, the bigger picture conjured by spirituality helps us cope with the setbacks thrown into the paths of our lives. It encourages contemplation and serves as a prescription to avoid the kind of knee-jerk reactions, or overreactions, that cause bigger problems than the one we were reacting to in the first place.
- **Self-awareness:** Spirituality helps us see ourselves as other people see us, steering us to view a problem or setback not just from the inside out but from the outside in. And from the outside, something we were fixated on may seem to be considerably less important than we had originally assessed. Too often we experience big

stress over small things because we see only ourselves in a group painting. Spirituality helps us widen the lens so we can better set our priorities.

- **Optimism:** Spirituality helps breed a positive outlook because it encourages us to believe something better and greater lies ahead. It keeps our focus trained forward instead of back, where we tend to relive things we've done and mistakes we've made that we'd do anything to change but can't. In that regard, I think about the character Rafiki from *The Lion King* continually smacking Simba in the head with his stick.

  "What'd you hit me for?" Simba asks him.

  "It doesn't matter. It's in the past," comes Rafiki's reply, which he follows with, "Oh yes, the past can hurt. But from the way I see it, you can either run from it or learn from it."

# OVERCOMING OBSTACLES

Overcoming obstacles is an essential part of life. Those obstacles teach us valuable lessons while helping to forge and define our character to achieve our highest potential. It's not something to be feared or avoided; instead, it should be embraced as a necessary part of personal growth and development.

Adversity is a part of life we all experience. It's safe to say that virtually all successful people got that way partly because they're adept at surmounting obstacles. Sometimes the degree to which we can overcome the debris life dumps in our path determines our very station in life. You can't avoid or escape obstacles thrown in the way of your journey. Too many, though, let those obstacles stop, define, or force them to backtrack and take a longer and more tedious route around such obstacles rather than overcoming them.

Overcoming obstacles is crucial to achieving success because it fosters resilience, builds character, teaches valuable life lessons, and develops essential skills like problem-solving and adaptability. The penchant reinforces that true achievement comes from navigating and learning from challenges rather than simply avoiding them; obstacles act as stepping stones on the path to success.[23]

And that produces the wider-ranging reality that the more you overcome in life, the more you value what you've attained. There are too many such obstacles to list, from health- and job-related issues to financial setbacks and relationships gone awry. Strategies and approaches to overcoming them are varied, and there's no one-size-fits-all formula. But there are some strategies you can employ in your daily life when faced with the need to surmount one of life's proverbial bumps in the road.

## PRESCRIPTIONS FOR OVERCOMING OBSTACLES

- **Acceptance:** Before surmounting an obstacle, you must acknowledge it's sitting right in front of you, blocking your path forward. Denial serves no one's best interests, because when you open your eyes again, it will still be there, no matter how much you wish it weren't.
- **Have a plan:** Don't wing it. If you try to jump over something without properly assessing it, you'll likely fail, and the toll on your mind and body makes success a much more challenging proposition. Having a plan will help you adapt if your strategy to surmount an incredibly stubborn obstacle comes up short initially.
- **Be willing to fail:** Running into an obstacle doesn't mean you've failed. You've only failed when you let that obstacle stop you in your tracks. Think about it. If you're driving somewhere and find the road ahead is closed, do you turn back or find another route? It may

take you longer to get where you're going, but you'll still get there. And every obstacle you overcome makes the next one less imposing and instills the confidence to know you can surmount it.

- **Take care of yourself:** The better your mental, emotional, and physical health, the better equipped you will be to deal with adversity of all kinds. The better you feel about yourself, the more resilient you will be, turning the obstacles ahead into bumps in the road instead of boulders.
- **Ask for help:** Just because you don't know how to get around what's blocking your chosen path doesn't mean somebody else won't. Others have traveled this same road before you and may be able to guide you around the obstacle in the manner they managed. Think about the world before navigation apps. You pulled into a gas station or asked a passerby for directions when you got lost. Those of us who failed to ask for help drove in circles before finally realizing we couldn't find the right path by ourselves.
- **Mentoring:** The largest pursuits bring the highest potential for setbacks and adversity. This is when you may need more than just help in the form of someone who can help chart a complete route for you instead of just one segment. This is especially true when starting a business or embarking on any bold new endeavor. It's easy to get discouraged, give up, or make predictable mistakes when taking on something for the first time. Starting that process by seeking out someone who's already done it can be an excellent strategy for

anticipating the obstacles likely to come up and preparing yourself to negotiate them successfully.

- **Therapy or counseling:** Psychotherapy can help you overcome obstacles by lending much-needed perspective and providing the tools your psyche needs to manage setbacks better. It can help patients recognize inaccurate or negative thoughts and how those thoughts affect the emotions and behaviors holding them back. It can also educate them on how to respond best when facing obstacles by establishing healthy coping strategies.

# PART THREE
## FINDING AND KEEPING HAPPINESS

*Most folks are as happy as they make up their minds to be.*

—ABRAHAM LINCOLN

*Not all patients come to me for treatment of a specific issue. Some come for mental health wellness check-ins, or just to talk, vent, or have a shoulder to cry on.*

*One such patient was a woman in her late forties who had a child with cerebral palsy. Having a disabled child can be a crushing burden for many, as I've seen firsthand in my practice. For this woman, though, it was a labor of love and a source of incredible joy for her.*

*The child was in their twenties at this point and showing signs of increasing decline normal for someone with CP. But that didn't faze my patient at all. She considered her child an incredible gift.*

*"My child is always, always happy. Never complains. And if they don't complain, how can I?"*

*My patient reveled in the fact that her child would always need her and remain an active and vital part of her life. She brought the child with her for a few sessions, and I was struck by the incredible love that existed between them, the kind of love you don't often see between parents and fully able children.*

*"Last year, my daughter and I decided to have breakfast in a different place every week. We kept a chart, like sticking pins in a map. It became like a mission. It was an example of knowing you're going to enjoy doing something and enjoy who you're doing it with. I wouldn't trade that for anything."*

*My patient had come to terms with a notion of child-rearing that the vast majority take for granted. Her attitude and perspective allowed her to find happiness and fulfillment in a thankless task that was only going to get harder.*

*One session, I told her how impressed I was and asked her what her secret was.*

*"The way my child smiles at me. No matter how I'm feeling, that smile makes it all worthwhile. My child is a ray of sunshine that brightens every day of my life."*

*She had found happiness and was never going to let go.*

# BECOMING AND STAYING HAPPY

A February 2024 survey by Gallup revealed only 47 percent of Americans consider themselves "very" satisfied with their lives, just a single point from the all-time record low.[24] While any number of factors have contributed to that alarming stat, one apparent reality emerges:

Less than half of this country is content with the state of their lives.

Over the years, I've asked new patients first, "What is it you want to get out of psychotherapy?" Although they all answer that question differently, it almost always boils down to the base desire to be happier than they are at present. Their current state, or prognosis, is often due to some upheaval they've experienced in their lives, an outside event like an accident or tragedy over which they had no control and that has claimed their happiness as a result.

I think better phrasing might be holding their happiness hostage, because my work frees them from that captivity by helping to identify the source of their unhappiness and providing potential options to lift them from their malaise. No one size fits all, but I've found a general rule when treating depression, for example, is to do a deep dive into the issues plaguing patients. If those issues are out of their control, like war or politics, I've found the key is for them to retrain their focus on what they can affect and where they can produce meaningful change. I might steer them into becoming an advocate for a cause they believe in, like the environment or homelessness. I might also suggest they discipline themselves to reduce the time they spend following the issue that is dragging them down. That could be as simple as watching a sporting event or movie or reading a book instead of a steady diet of cable news stations and social media. Leisure time should be just that.

I have seldom prescribed antidepressant drugs in my practice. While these drugs can produce miraculous results in some patients, they only mask the symptoms and often can create dependency. I prefer a different approach.

More often than we think, prevention really is worth a pound of cure. And when it comes to depression or general discontent with the state of your life, the more you proactively take care of your mental and physical health, the less likely life will drag you down and the more likely you'll be able to lift yourself back up when it does.

Bad things happen, and nobody will always be happy. Storm-proofing our lives is no different than preparing for the literal storms that can damage our homes instead of our psyches. So let's look at a few things you can do to maximize your chances of waking up every day feeling as good or better than the day before.

## PRESCRIPTIONS FOR BECOMING AND STAYING HAPPY

- **Focus:** The more time you spend doing what you enjoy with the people you enjoy being with, the happier you will be. Do less of what you feel you should and more of what you actually look forward to doing. Focusing on something good that's coming is a great way to keep a positive attitude.
- **Make somebody's day:** This could be as simple as saying thank you to someone or complimenting them on their work. Whatever it may be, making others feel good about themselves is a great recipe for feeling good about yourself. I have a patient, for example, who gives a dollar to every panhandler he meets because it reminds him of how much he has in his life by comparison. Keep a mental checklist, and at the end of the day, ask yourself how many people you helped, how many people had a better day because of you, and how many people you made smile or feel better about themselves.
- **Confront the bad:** Face your problems instead of avoiding or ignoring them, which only allows them to fester. The more you make believe something bad isn't there, the more likely it will get worse. That means dealing with issues proactively when it's still early, instead of reactively when it's often too late.
- **Positivity:** Surround yourself with the people who make you feel better about yourself and avoid those who produce the opposite effect. Negativity is never a good thing, and the more you can avoid conflict and

unpleasantness, the happier you will be. "When I find myself stuck in a pattern of negative thinking," wrote Dr. Kali D. Cyrus, a psychiatrist and assistant professor at Johns Hopkins University School of Medicine, for *The New York Times*, "I try not to complain for seven days. It retrains your brain to stop going down a negative path. I write, 'Don't complain!' on a sticky note right by my bed so I can see it when I wake up."[25]

- **Look in the mirror:** I've had too many patients over the years who, initially anyway, judge themselves in comparison to others. You can only be the best *you*, not the best version of someone else.

# NEW PURSUITS AND INTERESTS

I've learned firsthand that part of healthy aging is undertaking new pursuits and interests. Ten years ago, I became an ordained rabbi, which required a substantial investment in time and study. The process made me feel like a college or medical student again, which was the point of pursuing something I'd always thought passionately about. I never said or thought I was too old, that the opportunity to do something I always dreamed of had passed me by. Dreams, as long as they're not something too physically taxing or unrealistic, don't change, and we're never too old to pursue them.

More recently, I decided to invest another considerable amount of time and passion to write this book. I might be seeing fewer patients these days and doing it almost exclusively through Zoom, but I've lost none of my interest in or passion for the field of mental health. This book represents the fulfillment of another dream for me in that it has captured much of my life and work experience to share with those I cannot treat personally. No psychiatrist can treat thousands of people at once in their practice, but with this book, I can reach far more people than all the patients I've seen in my lifetime practicing psychiatry.

Often, a person will find the passion for a new pursuit or interest outside of how they've spent the bulk of their lives. There's no reason, for example, why a high school graduate who's just retired from their chosen trade can't work toward a degree at a local state or community college at very low tuition. Should they choose, the person could then parlay that into teaching classes, either as a substitute at the public school level or to fellow adults at the community school level.

I have a client who's built a career as a successful writer. Recently, that client started teaching for a local program where anyone can sign up for a small fee. He told me recently that the bulk of his students are older than forty, and most are closer to sixty or even beyond. In that respect, he's getting as much from the experience as his students are. Call it a win-win.

A retired librarian might think out of the box and opt to take classes in landscape design. A retired English teacher whose life has been defined by a love of books might get a job at a bookstore. A former college baseball player who was always too busy to coach his son's Little League team can get a second bite at that apple by coaching his grandchild's team—all examples of a win-win.

To that end, I've had patients who've pursued what they thought were only hobbies that ultimately developed into second careers. I had another patient who loved flowers more than anything. When time and opportunity finally allowed, he took classes in botany that morphed into a second career in floriculture, the branch of horticulture that focuses on the cultivation, marketing, and arrangement of flowers and ornamental plants.

I haven't seen him in a while, but on one of our last visits, he told me he was happier than he's ever been in his life.

## PRESCRIPTIONS FOR NEW PURSUITS AND INTERESTS

- **Mental stimulation:** Learning new skills presents new challenges for the mind and the body. You may have heard the phrase "use it or lose it" at some point. Nothing is healthier mentally and spiritually than trying something new to break out of a rut or a by-the-numbers routine that leaves you unfulfilled.
- **Emotional health:** Nothing makes us feel better than succeeding at something new. It does wonders for our self-esteem, and the importance of feeling good about ourselves does not diminish with age. Here's a prescription for happiness: waking up every morning looking forward to at least one thing you're going to do that day.
- **Engagement:** New endeavors mean meeting new people and offering a chance to bolster your social circle with new friends with whom you enjoy a shared interest. In that regard, maintaining a sense of community is another prescription for happiness. Time alone can be great, but pervasive social isolation demeans your quality of life.
- **Physical health:** Taking on something new goes to the heart of the mind-body connection. Even if your new pursuit isn't something like pickleball, tennis, or some form of physical endeavor, your improved sense of well-being is just what the doctor ordered for your

overall health. And the better you feel, the more active you will be.

- **Personal growth:** I've had so many older patients who tell me they feel like they're floundering because every day feels the same. The problem is I've found too often that stagnation leads to decline. So I'll frequently ask my patients suffering from this proclivity to tell me something they've never done but would still love to do. One told me he always wanted to fly a plane. My response to him was, "What are you waiting for?"

# CONFLICT RESOLUTION

I've never had a patient who enjoys or revels in conflict. Avoiding conflict, as well as learning how best to cope with the inevitability of it, is an excellent prescription for finding and keeping happiness.

I talk to patients about empowering themselves by not overreacting to conflict or, in some cases, not reacting at all. Someone might say something to you that's unpleasant, inaccurate, or even hurtful. You won't win an argument with that person or achieve anything by confronting them. We're told from the time we're children to walk away from a fight. The same holds for avoiding conflict by turning your back on someone trying to engage you that way.

This is especially true these days, thanks to our fractured political climate. I can't tell you how many patients I have who've cut off contact with friends and even close relatives because they disagree, often vehemently, on politics. I'll ask them what they liked the most about this other person before conflict ruled the day. After they answer me, I ask, "Well, isn't that still the case?" I know how annoying it can be when someone wears their opinions on their sleeve and sticks them in your face. But you have the right to turn away and ignore those opinions and focus on who they are instead. Empower yourself by not giving them the fight they want.

Conflict and strife often appear in emails and texts for many of my patients. People tend to type words they'd never say to you out loud, and you must take them in that context. Don't respond right away, when the feeling is still raw and you're seething. If your dander is up, write your response, but don't send it. That's why the Drafts folder is one of the greatest inventions of electronic communication. Blow off whatever steam you need to by getting your own angry words down, but make a rule for yourself not to send the message for twenty-four hours, after you've had a chance to cool off a bit. Then reread your email and see if it's something you still want to send. Sometimes, the best response is no response at all.

Commit right now to doing this with the next three contentious messages you receive and see how much better you feel by avoiding the conflict altogether. When you ultimately reengage with the person and explain your reaction calmly, they'll inevitably say something like, "That's not what I meant at all." I can't tell you how many friendships and relationships between family members have been grievously harmed by saying something you can never take back in writing. Misunderstandings and miscommunication represent a prime root cause of conflict.

The tendency to overreact roils us all, as does a growing trend I've observed in my practice of people losing perspective. Recently, I watched a segment on television featuring a well-known and respected psychiatrist preaching the mantra that if you don't get along with family members, don't spend the holidays with them. Just avoid the conflict entirely. That sounds ridiculous, given the more positive prescriptions I've already offered. You shouldn't avoid a situation out of concern over what someone might say. If you let them push your buttons, you're as guilty as they are for allowing that to happen. You need to be the adult in the room, because your relative is at the kiddie table. If you avoid spending the holiday with such a person out of fear of what they might say, they emerge as the victor in a conflict you didn't even engage in.

## PRESCRIPTIONS FOR CONFLICT RESOLUTION

- **Find common ground:** Forget about bridging the gap between you. Focus instead on areas you have in common. Favorite sports teams, for example, or relatives the two of you are equally endeared to. Next time you're out at a family function or other gathering, make a mental note whenever you don't clash with someone who says or does something that leaves you shaking your head or reaching for your car keys.
- **Open and honest communication:** It's easy to preach this but difficult to practice, because we don't live in a perfect world. Listening to the other person's perspective is probably not as effective a strategy as not listening at all or finding something else to talk about where neither of you is trying to sway the other to their way of thinking, because that's not going to happen. We're all set in our ways, so don't bother trying to change anyone's opinion or engage with anyone who's trying to change yours.
- **First person:** Saying "I feel" or "I think" is a great way to avoid conflict, because you're not making a definitive

statement so much as offering your thoughts. There's a difference between making absolute pronouncements you can't back up and stating how you feel about something because of a particular experience. Again, this requires you to be the adult in the room, and when someone says something offensive that angers or annoys you, that's the time to find a reason to leave the table.

- **Converse, don't argue:** Sure, you can ask open-ended questions to gain a deeper understanding of the other person's viewpoint, but chances are they're not going to respond in kind. Again, the issue isn't how you put anything—it's what you choose to talk about in the first place. There's a national gym chain that has what's called a "Lunk Alarm," which goes off when someone grunts, groans, or drops the weights. All gatherings should have a Conflict Alarm that activates when someone decides to pontificate on something no one else wants to hear about, much less argue over.
- **Choose your battles:** Sometimes, someone says something so ludicrous and offensive that you feel you must respond. That's natural, it's human. But know where that line is drawn for you, and only react when it's crossed.
- **Empathy:** I can't stress this enough, because sometimes when someone is absurdly vociferous about something, it's because something else is going on in their lives that has stolen their perspective. Be sensitive to people's feelings and emotions, and don't be the person who lashes out at someone whose behavior is rooted in a recent loss or downturn they've been carrying around with them.

# MANAGING STRESS

Stress and conflict are often viewed as interchangeable. They are not. Far from it. You can walk away from conflict, but you can't walk away from stress. Some stress is inevitable. It's an indelible part of our lives, and how well we manage it goes a long way toward determining the level of happiness we can maintain.

Things happen that cause you anxiety, those moments in life that steal your sleep and dominate your waking hours. Unlike avoiding conflict, they are things that are either out of your control or something within your control that went badly. An example of the former is losing your job because of downsizing. An example of the latter is losing money in a bad investment. Either way, you cannot change what happened, only how you react to it.

How you handle and process stress is up to you. I've seen far too many people display the proclivity of either running from the problem by ignoring it, digging themselves a deeper hole to fall into, or losing perspective by letting the situation dominate their lives. All these are counterproductive, and far too often, stress takes its toll on the body by weakening the immune system and often manifesting in digestion-related symptoms. That means part of managing stress is knowing how to manage its physical effects, for which Dr. Lin Chang, a gastroenterologist at UCLA, offers one practical solution.

"Diaphragmatic breathing—using your diaphragm to take deep, controlled breaths and expand your belly, followed by exhaling slowly and letting your belly fall—stimulates vagus nerve activity and potentially reduces gastrointestinal symptoms such as bloating. I do it at bedtime for about 10 minutes."[26]

Let's look at some other productive and proactive ways to respond to stress.

## PRESCRIPTIONS FOR MANAGING STRESS

- **Pets:** There's a good reason cats and dogs are brought to visit hospitals, schools, and veterans centers. Interacting with animals can decrease levels of the stress hormone cortisol and even lower your blood pressure. Just by being in their company, pets can have a remarkably positive effect on us, perhaps because they imbue us with responsibility that reminds us of our more significant priorities.[27] That said, caring for pets isn't for everyone, and there are other ways to reduce stress that you don't have to feed.
- **Avoid information overload:** When stressed, our plates are full. The last thing we need is to add more peripheral stress by surfing social media in search of relief, a quest more likely to result in further agitation. Being under stress makes for an opportune time to reduce incoming stimuli in favor of distractions like

a sporting event or concert. Avoid contact with those who aren't anything but a positive influence on you, in whose company you feel better, and who make you feel better about yourself, which is what you need to handle what's already on your plate.

- **Maintain perspective:** There's a reason why the old adage "don't sweat the little stuff" has stood the test of time. We spend way too much energy stressing over things that don't really amount to much. Many of us also tend to fixate on things either out of our control or what we shouldn't be bothering ourselves about in the first place. Sometimes, too, you must put distance between yourself and those dragging you down or holding you back. If the stress concerns a loved one's illness, focus on the treatment that will make them well again. And if you can't be as strong for yourself as you like, be strong for them, which can serve as therapy for you. I don't ordinarily recommend comparisons as therapy, but sometimes considering how fortunate you are to have what you've got, compared to others who are in far more dire straits, can be a prescription for minimizing the effects of stress.
- **Compartmentalize:** This goes to the old cliché: Don't bring your work home. By the same token, don't bring your home to your work. It's not only practical to segment your life this way. This practice also helps you better cope with stress, because distancing yourself from it, however briefly, is a positive prescription too. As hard as it may seem, try to keep stress confined to the part of your life where it originated, and try not to

drag it with you elsewhere—a tall order, I know, but one that will be well worth the effort.

- **A good night's sleep:** Yet another cliché comes into play here: "Sleep on it, and you'll feel better about things in the morning." That's not just an old saying; it's actually true. When you sleep, your mind keeps working, and you may well awaken with a fresh perspective on, or a new solution for, what's plaguing you. Unfortunately, the reverse is also the case, as tossing and turning all night to fixate on things will only exacerbate your stress level.
- **Don't self-medicate:** Speaking of sleep, I never recommend sleep aids for this kind of predicament, because they alter the sleep cycle and can be counterproductive. So, too, you can't drink yourself out of a problem with alcohol or swallow yourself out of a problem with antianxiety medication. That just dulls the pain, and when your self-prescribed answer wears off, you'll find yourself worse off than before.
- **Exercise:** I may sound like a broken record regarding exercise as a cure-all for everything that ails us, but that isn't far from the truth. Forcing the body and mind to work together on a physical pursuit of your choice is a great way to separate yourself from stress and thus face the cause through a different lens and clearer head. Too many people under stress break their normal routine of working out because they can't focus on anything else but what is dominating their lives. That is when you need to prioritize exercise and other pursuits even more.
- **Mental exercises:** When dealing with stress, these can be just as important as the physical variety. As in many

treatments, you need to find what works best for you. Dr. Aditi Nerurkar, a Harvard physician specializing in stress and burnout, offers one she calls Stop, Breathe, Be, which "is a three-second brain reset to help manage anxiety in the moment. The instructions are in the name: Stop whatever you're doing, take a brief pause. Take a deep breath in and out. Be grounded in the present moment. 'Stop, Breathe, Be' gets you out of 'What if?' thinking and back to what is, in the here and now."[28]

- **Ask for help:** No person is an island, yet another old saying goes, and this is as on point as it gets when you're under stress. If the stress is constant, shifting almost continuously from one issue to the next, it may be time to consider seeing a professional who can provide an objective view. Alternatively, this may also be the time to seek out those you know who will tell you like it is instead of what you want to hear. Don't expect them to have the magic answer you're looking for, but if something they say points you in the right direction, that's good enough.

# ENVY AND JEALOUSY

A few pages back, I noted that, according to Gallup, less than half of all Americans, 47 percent, report being "very satisfied" with their lives.[29] So it's no wonder that up to 53 percent of the population are likely to find themselves envying those who have what they don't and jealous of them for it. Envy and jealousy can act like a self-destruct switch on a person's emotional well-being. You can disable the switch—or make reaching for it an afterthought—only by becoming more satisfied with who you are and your station in life, and that process starts by addressing your self-esteem.

Self-esteem is a term that gets thrown around a lot with regard to children, but adults need to maintain theirs just as much as kids do. We all have ways of enhancing it throughout our lives: by the relationships we choose, our work, our families, our dedication to causes, or the community we've surrounded ourselves with. The stronger these pillars of our lives are, the less we will subject ourselves to being envious or jealous of someone who we perceive has more than we do.

The key to happiness, many would say, is to celebrate what you have in life and not fixate on what you don't. You tend not to think the grass is greener on the other side when you're perfectly content with the landscaping on your side. I've treated many patients who fixate on what they don't have and spend our session telling me about a neighbor, friend, or co-worker who has a better life than they do. "Really?" I say to them. "If they looked at you, tell me something they would say you have in your life that's better." Almost inevitably, the patient comes up with a whole litany of things that I then use to make them see their lives differently. You can only be the best person you can be, not the best person you think somebody else is.

Envy or jealousy actually has more to do with us than whoever we're comparing ourselves to. It often shows up in my patients who've lost confidence in themselves and don't feel they're as good at things as they used to be or even not good at anything anymore. Maybe they sold the business that long defined their identity. Maybe their kids have grown up and moved on, denying them the paternal or maternal sense that overrode everything else for years. Even at a relatively young age, in their mid to late forties or early fifties, they feel lost because everyone they know seems to be in a better place and station in life. They've lost their ability to feel good about themselves and be confident in their approach to everything. So what's the prescription for them?

It starts with asking a patient who's come to see me, "Why do you feel that way now?" And they might say, "Well, I've been feeling it for ten years, but I finally decided to do something about it." Okay, let's do something about it. Let's try to figure out what happened and what changed. Has this been a recurring theme in your life, or is it something new? Might it be the result of some kind of trauma you suffered?

It's our nature to envy others and be jealous of their achievements or accomplishments. That shouldn't mean you don't appreciate what you have, and there's nothing wrong with wanting more or emulating someone who has it. What's wrong is when you are constantly comparing yourself to others and obsessed with what's missing from your life instead of focusing on what's present in it.

Here are some strategies to avoid falling into the trap of envy and jealousy.

## PRESCRIPTIONS FOR AVOIDING ENVY AND JEALOUSY

- **Look in the mirror:** Train your focus on yourself, not others, by celebrating what you've already achieved and look forward to achieving. In that respect, instead of being envious or jealous of someone, use them as an example or role model by seeking to attain whatever you feel they have that you don't. In the case of money or possessions, though, don't seek what others have, because your needs are different. Set your expectations and goals based on you, not somebody else.
- **Coping mechanisms:** We've already mentioned the old saying about the grass being greener on the other side. The problem is that sometimes the metaphorical fence is so tall you can't tell if the grass is real or artificial. Too often we lose perspective and don't look below the surface to see if the person we are envious of is really happy. You may want something they have, but

ask yourself if, given the chance, you'd actually like to switch places with them.

- **Avoid negativity:** Comparing ourselves to others invites negative thoughts because we inherently focus on what they may have and we don't. Ask yourself what *you* have that the person you're jealous of doesn't.
- **Be a cheerleader:** Life is neither a competition nor a zero-sum game proposition. No one must fail for you to succeed, so celebrate the successes of friends or acquaintances. That attitude is one I see all the time in the most successful of my patients. They not only root for others to win, but they will also aid a friend or relative in that task. The happier you are when others triumph, the more likely you are to triumph yourself.
- **Develop your self-worth:** A person is far more than the measure of their possessions or what they have attained in life. And I can tell you from treating a slew of very wealthy and successful people that their financial and material worth often barely makes up for how unhappy they are about their lives. People should measure themselves by who they are, not what they have.

# PRACTICING GRATITUDE

I've gotten myself into a place where in the morning, if I start having bad thoughts upon waking up, I say, *Stop that! Be grateful that you're getting up, that you're feeling pretty good, and that you've got a great day ahead of you.* Similarly, when I go to bed, I get myself into a place of gratitude for what I have achieved throughout the day. Who did I help? Who did I make feel better about themselves? What did I do to feel better about myself? I firmly believe that practicing gratitude is key to achieving and maintaining happiness.

Not enough emphasis is given to the positive effects of just saying "thank you" or "good job." I have an exercise for you to perform: For one week, keep a running tally in your mind of how many people ahead of you in checkout lines say thank you to the person who rang up and bagged their groceries or other purchases. Do you thank the bank teller for depositing or cashing your check? Do you thank the mailman for delivering your mail? How often do you thank someone for just doing their job? It makes their day more fulfilling when you do, and here's the thing: It produces the same effect on you.

The simplest gestures can go a long way. Many toil in obscurity, doing their best, with little attention ever paid to their effort or accomplishment. I don't think we understand how valuable recognition is to them and to us for providing it. Practicing gratitude is the bailiwick of a person with a more expansive view of the world before and around them. They notice things others don't and are further enriched and thus happy because of it.

I have another exercise for you to try: For the next ten days, I want you to say "thank you" to someone at least three times a day. You'll be amazed at your opportunities when you expand the lens through which you see the world. For now, ask yourself when you last thanked someone for doing only what was expected of them.

Here are some ways to practice the simple act of expressing your gratitude as a prescription for happiness.

## PRESCRIPTIONS FOR PRACTICING GRATITUDE

- **What goes around, comes around:** Nobody gets more out of complimenting someone else than you. Making someone feel better about themselves bears a direct correlation to you feeling better about yourself.
- **A wider lens:** Showing gratitude means retraining your focus through a wider lens, encouraging you to see things you may have missed before. It helps us understand that sometimes, the simplest things yield the greatest reward and pleasure.

- **Self-esteem:** Viewing the world with a sense of gratitude can change how you think about your worth. Think about how good it makes you feel when you go to lunch or dinner with a friend and they pick up the tab. As you express your appreciation, you also realize that your friend is spending time and resources on you because you're important to them. And maybe the next time you're out with a different friend, you pick up the tab instead.
- **Enhanced patience:** The more you thank people, the less likely you are to be short with them when doing their best isn't enough for you. You might just be having a bad day, but practicing gratitude regularly makes you less likely to lash out at some clerk, tech, or phone rep whose performance may be frustrating you. You don't want to ruin their day any more than you want someone to ruin yours.
- **Make someone's day:** I have found the more I try to make someone's day, the more they strive to make mine the next time I'm in their checkout line or being served by them in a restaurant or need to visit the auto repair shop in an emergency. Being nice almost invariably raises you in the esteem of others, and they will want to make your day whenever they can, just as you made theirs.

# ACCEPTANCE

Accepting your lot in life does not mean you're completely satisfied and won't continue trying to improve your standing. Acceptance is necessary for self-improvement, since the alternative is bemoaning your situation and being preoccupied with the negative instead of the positive. Acceptance builds a platform off which you can continue to grow, because it implies focusing on the positive (what you do have) instead of the negative (what you don't).

A lot of people begin psychotherapy because they want to be happier. They don't express acceptance of the life they have and may talk a lot about what their lives are lacking. They may complain about having a child who's never amounted to anything. I'll ask them to tell me something good about that son or daughter, and they'll say something like, "Oh, they're such a talented artist but haven't managed to make a living at it yet." I try to get that patient to accept their child for who they are, a precursor for getting the patient to accept themselves as they are at the same time.

Being more accepting of yourself encourages you to be more accepting of others and, thus, less critical of them. That's an important point I can't stress enough, because a portion of our mental health consists of a series of circles. In this case, accepting yourself means better accepting others, and accepting others makes you more likely to be less critical of yourself.

There's nothing wrong with wanting to be better. In that respect, acceptance should not be confused with complacency or laziness. You're not saying, *I accept that this is all I will ever be*. Instead, you're saying, *I like where I am, but next year at this time, I want to love where I am.* There is no better predictor for unhappiness than perpetual disgruntlement with the state of your life, because it could indicate that you will never be satisfied with what you have. Life will be nothing more than a race for more; ultimately, it's a race everyone with that attitude loses.

Having trouble with acceptance? Consider the following.

## PRESCRIPTIONS FOR ACCEPTANCE

- **A temporary state:** Nobody stays on top forever, and the reverse of that is an attitude that everyone should adopt. Believe in your heart that challenging times are transitory and that you're working toward what lies on the other side. If you believe the negative dominates your life, it will continue to dominate it until you make room for the positive.
- **Self-criticism:** We tend to be hard on ourselves, holding ourselves to a higher and potentially unrealistic standard. Think about how accepting you are of other people, warts and all. Then why are you continually so critical of yourself? There's nothing wrong with having high expectations, but there's a lot wrong with beating

yourself up over not meeting those expectations every single time.

- **"You got this":** That's what someone says to us to boost our confidence or make us feel better about ourselves. I don't think we say it to ourselves enough. Believing you can do something is the first step to getting it done. In that regard, I can't stress enough how important it is not to accept failure in advance. *I can't do this because I failed the last time* versus *I know where I came up short last time*. There's a massive difference between those disparate attitudes, and attitude when it comes to acceptance is everything.
- **Don't overthink:** We are all prone to this. No one ever emerges better for turning a problem into a battle or a battle into a war, usually with ourselves over the inability to accept something at face value. Overcomplicating things can be a serious impediment to our capacity to accept.
- **Carrying a grudge:** So, too, we often find ourselves carrying grudges, refusing to accept another's behavior toward us, or blowing that behavior out of proportion. It's not as simple as if you want to be happy, don't carry any grudges. But the more grudges you carry, the less happy you will be. It's better to move on, grin, and bear it. I have a patient who says of people who've wronged him, "They're off the list!" This means that they've been excised from that person's life. And banishing someone is better for your happiness because you've removed the burden they had become.
- **A lower standard:** The more you expect from people, the more likely they will disappoint you. In that

respect, holding them to a lower standard means you will more easily accept them. Perhaps you have trouble accepting your stake in life because you hold yourself to such a high standard that you've set expectations for yourself that cannot be met. I'm not advocating for you to aim lower or practice less ambition. If you regard yourself objectively rather than subjectively, though, you may find there is far more to celebrate and accept than bemoaning the lack thereof.

# MODERATION

There's a reason why we hear the adage "everything in moderation" so frequently repeated. Because it's true!

Much of psychiatry is about helping patients find a balance between the extremes that often plague them. Moderation is crucial to happiness because it allows for a balanced approach to life and avoids the consequences of resorting to extremes, the result of that being greater overall satisfaction and well-being. Essentially, "everything in moderation" helps you maintain a healthy and happy lifestyle.

Often, that phrase is thought to refer only to the consumption of food and drink. But the same principle holds for many other parts of our lives. Being an alcoholic is bad for you, but so can being a workaholic. Being an involved parent can be great until you become overbearing and start berating officials who didn't call a foul that caused your child to miss a shot.

It all comes down to striking a balance. Keeping things in moderation sharpens our perspective, and happiness is easier to find and keep when our perspective is clear. I'd like to stress that many of the patients who come to see me—and I suspect many of you reading this book—aren't as happy as they once were. I refuse to accept that as a natural progression of life. I will say, though, that as our lives change, so must our perspectives. You can't look at life at forty or sixty through the same lens you did at twenty. That may seem like an extreme example, but it's easy to lose yourself when you're not framing your life in the proper context. When I treat people suffering from that, my first goal is to reframe their lives based on where they are now, not where they were or want to be.

Let's look at some strategies to actively and consciously practice moderation.

## PRESCRIPTIONS FOR PRACTICING MODERATION

- **Avoid burnout:** Running is great for you, but if you run every day, you could harm yourself physically to the point you'll never run again. The same holds true for just about everything. Trainers advise lifting weights every other day to allow the body to recover. I tell patients to always look forward to getting back to what they love to do. If you overdo what you love, you risk losing your passion for it. Instead, maintain your passion by practicing moderation.
- **Stability:** Moderation is the best way to maintain balance in life, and that balance will serve your state of happiness well. Extreme highs give way to equally extreme lows, which makes happiness elusive because you're constantly chasing what you lost instead of enjoying and celebrating what you have. That's the very definition of despair.

- **Relationships:** Maintaining balance in relationships with friends and loved ones is perhaps the most essential basis for retaining happiness or finding it again if you've lost it. The people in your life are your rocks. They create the stability you need to keep your life steady. The old saying that "a strong ship can weather any storm" may not be true literally, but it is true figuratively because you need to be able to withstand life's storms so you can emerge happy again when those storms pass. There's another old adage that "people keep you humble." And it's humility that will help you keep things in moderation.
- **Fitness:** As I've said before, exercise and diet should be a foundation of your life to maintain or restore happiness. So, too, practicing moderation in diet and exercise is key to maintaining good physical health, significantly impacting happiness.
- **Self-awareness:** It's important to view yourself objectively, as others see you. It's not a matter of doing things to please and make people think better of you; it's a matter of consistency so they know what to expect from you. When you're self-aware, you can police your tendencies to swing too high and too low. It's important to note that in some cases, mood swings are the result of psychological issues like bipolar disorder, which require treatment and medication to restore the body's natural balance. But they don't make a pill to keep us in moderation otherwise. We have to rely on our psyches for that.

# PART FOUR
# COPING WITH TRAUMA

*Character cannot be developed in ease and quiet. Only through experience of trial and suffering can the soul be strengthened, ambition inspired, and success achieved.*

—HELEN KELLER

*A long-time patient came to see me because he'd suffered one of the truly worst tragedies imaginable: the death of his son at the hands of a drunk driver in a car accident.*

*"I don't want to get out of bed in the morning. I can't think of anything else other than my boy. I'm not sure I even want to go on living."*

*I've probably seen more patients over trauma than anything else. The lingering nature of trauma symptoms is often the impetus behind the appointment requests I get from patients both old and new. They figure things will get better with time and call me when the effects linger beyond their expectations. Their first question, inevitably, is, "When will I feel better?" That's an impossible question to answer, because no two people's timetables are the same. People heal on the inside at different paces, just as they heal in the same fashion on the outside.*

*I didn't tell that father not to feel the way he did, because that's what he needed to feel in that moment. In our first session, I didn't even ask him about the son he had tragically lost. Instead, I asked him all about his other two kids—not just how they were coping with the loss, but what they had done in their lives that made him the proudest. He shined as he described their accomplishments, what made them special too, and I sensed this was the first time he had spoken about anything other than his late son in the weeks since the young man's death.*

*I did this to get him to focus on the pillars of his life that were still standing, and, on his own, he expressed how he needed to be strong for them even when he couldn't be strong for himself. In our next session, we focused on his wife. And the week after we delved into my patient's relationship with his own parents and how he learned to be a father.*

*Nothing I could say would make the pain go away, so I focused instead on numbing it as best I could by bringing to light all my patient still had to be grateful for in his life. He'll never get over the loss of his son but he was able to view it in a different light. And by the time I felt the time was right to focus on his son, he was more prone to celebrate the young man than mourn him. I made the point of telling him he could do both and that following such a prescription, along with being strong for his surviving children and wife, was the best way he could find his purpose in life again.*

# OVERCOMING GRIEF

The longer you're lucky enough to live, the more you will experience the death of acquaintances, friends, and loved ones. That's a fact of life, and we can do nothing to change it.

Make no mistake about it: Grief can take a terrible toll on a person's physical health as well as their emotional well-being. "People who are depressed often isolate themselves and withdraw from social connections and they often stop taking care of themselves properly," Dr. Maureen Malin explained to Harvard Health Publishing. "You're not as interested in life. You fall down on the job, miss doctor appointments, stop exercising, stop eating properly. All of these things put your health at risk."[30]

It's especially hard the first time you lose someone close to you. I'd like to say you get used to it, that it becomes easier to bear, but that's not true. Each of us needs to grieve a loss in our own way—there are no absolutes and no one-size-fits-all prescribed remedies. Your life will go on. You may cycle through some or all of the long-accepted five stages of grief—denial, anger, bargaining, depression, and acceptance—but you will do so in an order that fits who you are. There's no one good way to overcome grief, and it's often a combination of factors that lifts you from the morass of loss.

The first and most important thing to realize is that grief is a natural phenomenon. The end of life is a part of life, even when that end comes earlier than expected and sometimes suddenly. When someone you're close to, even love, passes away, you will experience a wide range of emotions, whether the death was anticipated or not. Many people initially feel numb upon hearing the news, but like physical pain, the (heart)ache sets in once the numbness subsides.

We tend to live our lives within a relatively narrow band of emotions. We can do just fine until something as severe as grief forces us out of our lane into what the new reality of profound loss leaves us with. The process of grieving is all about finding your way back to normalcy, to the point where your life starts to resemble the way it was before the dreaded phone call informing you of the news came. You can't escape that reality by not answering the phone any more than you can set out on the road to recovery until you progress naturally through a wide range of emotions that range from shock to despair, from denial to confusion, from sadness to acceptance. These emotions are natural and common reactions to loss. You might be surprised by how intense your feelings are, how long they last, or how quickly your mood shifts. It's not uncommon to question your mental stability, but rest assured, these responses are a normal part of coming to terms with your loss.

Here's a coping mechanism to combat that from Sherry Cormier, a psychologist and bereavement trauma expert: "A couple times a day, I consciously drop my shoulders, sigh, and think to myself, 'Let's go.'"[31]

There is no one, single prescription for overcoming grief, but there are strategies that can help you cope with your loss and minimize the time the resulting despair dominates your life.

## PRESCRIPTIONS FOR OVERCOMING GRIEF

- **Commiserate with others:** Don't bear your grief alone. Seek solace in the company of others who share the pain of your loss. Instead of just mourning who you have lost, seek to celebrate their life with stories and shared experiences. Start your sentences with some version of "Remember when he or she…" because that helps you cherish the memories you have of the person. You can't get that person back, but you can keep them close in your mind and your heart.
- **Open up:** A big part of working through the grieving process is not holding your feelings in. It's like blowing up a balloon—sooner or later, it pops. You need to express your feelings, not turn them inward, where you risk losing yourself in the hole you're digging. This is one of those times when psychotherapy is recommended if you lack a suitable alternative outlet. When I have patients come to me because they're grieving, I encourage them to take what they miss most about who they've lost and put it into action. Lend your support to a cause that was important to them. Watch the team you both rooted for play. Strategic coping means finding positive ways to grieve that lift you from your doldrums.

- **Take care of your physical health:** So many patients I've treated who were grieving stopped eating right and exercising. When I ask them why, the standard answer is, "I just don't feel like it right now. Why bother?" Early on, I give them a pass. Fairly quickly, though, I urge them to push themselves back into a healthy routine. Coping with grief emotionally and mentally requires us not to neglect ourselves physically.
- **Move forward:** Notice I didn't say move *on*. These are two wholly disparate reactions. Getting stuck in the moment of grief means being frozen in time. You don't advance, grow, or progress, which are the primary ingredients of life at any age. You can move forward with your life as you grieve. You don't have to wait to stop grieving to do that, and you shouldn't.
- **Be patient:** Nobody heals on the outside the same way, and the same holds true for the inside. Give yourself time. It's okay to be sad for a while. What isn't okay is allowing sadness to consume your life.
- **Be strong for others:** Taking on the responsibility of checking in or looking after others who share your loss can be a great way to cope with grief. Helping others is one of the strongest prescriptions for strong mental and emotional health in the broadest sense. Similarly, if you can help someone grieving the same loss, you will help yourself in the process.
- **Cherish the day:** Strive to never leave anything on the table in your most important relationships. Never think you'll have time tomorrow to make a call, make plans, or make changes you should be making today. With my patients, I've found the greatest impediment

to recovering from grief is regret. Losing someone close can leave you mourning not only them but also what you didn't do when you had a chance. Living a life with as few regrets as possible is a strong recipe for coping with any kind of trauma.

- **Psychotherapy:** Seeing a professional can reap great benefits for someone experiencing grief. It's one of the primary reasons why patients come to see me, for the toll grief is taking on the quality of their lives. It can make even the simplest tasks difficult and can also make finding joy in anything nearly impossible. A psychotherapist can help put things in the proper perspective so the patient learns to weigh the experience against the totality of their lives, instead of letting the effects of grief define, dominate, and overshadow everything else.

# DEALING WITH ILLNESS OR INFIRMITY

Physical decline is inevitable, but its pace and detrimental effects, to a fairly large degree, are within your control. You can cheat Father Time for longer than you think if you exercise properly and eat right.

As it turns out, other mental health experts are playing that same record. A study published in *The Journals of Gerontology*, as reported by AARP, reported that "research reinforces a life-span approach to maintaining physical ability—don't wait until you are 80 years old and cannot get out of a chair," lead author Katherine Hall, assistant professor of medicine at Duke, advances. "The good news is, the ability to function independently can often be preserved with regular exercise."[32]

A 2024 study by Statista found that 60 percent of American adults are afraid to face the effects of aging.[33] A 2014 study from the pharmaceutical giant Pfizer revealed that a staggering 87 percent of those surveyed fear getting older, especially the physical decline that comes with it.[34] So why did a relatively low percentage of them say they exercise regularly? There's a reason why the Fountain of Youth has remained such an enduring myth. People forever fantasize about some magical pill or potion that will reverse the effects of aging or, at the very least, stop or slow the process.

You know what? It already exists.

There is no better prescription for maximizing your quality and quantity of life than eating right and finding a workout regimen that works for you. I've had patients who've given up on both as they age, offering the familiar refrain, "What's the difference? At my age, it doesn't matter anymore." Well, yes, it does, more than ever, actually. So, too, when I ask patients how they're taking care of themselves, I've heard too often, "I can't work out anymore." I urge them to change their expectations. If you can't run a mile, walk it. If you can't lift the weight you used to, switch to another program that makes you use resistance bands or another suitable alternative. A recent National Institutes of Health report found, "Laboratory-based studies showed that 20 to 30 minutes of strength (resistance) training, 2 to 3 times per week, has positive effects on risk factors for cardiovascular disorders, cancer, diabetes, and osteoporosis."[35]

My point being that diet and exercise are the closest things we have to that Fountain of Youth.

Let's explore other ways to ward off illness and infirmity for as long as mentally and physically possible.

## PRESCRIPTIONS FOR DEALING WITH ILLNESS OR INFIRMITY

- **Meditation:** This can be like exercise for the mind, helping you place your thoughts in the proper perspective.

Meditation can positively impact your outlook on life by reducing stress and anxiety, enhancing emotional regulation, increasing self-awareness, promoting a more positive mindset, fostering resilience in the face of challenges, and allowing you to view situations with greater clarity and perspective, leading to a more optimistic outlook on life.[36]

- **Don't self-medicate:** Seniors are abusing alcohol as a coping mechanism for their perceived decline in increasing numbers.[37] But having two glasses of wine every night instead of one or drinking earlier in the day out of boredom or low spirits serves only to exacerbate the issues that led you to drink, or abuse other "remedies," in the first place. According to a 2016 study reported on practicalneurology.com, "Men who consumed 36 grams/day of alcohol experienced a *faster 10-year decline* in all cognitive domains."[38]
- **Avoid antidepressants:** A disturbing trend I've noted as of late is older patients asking me to prescribe antidepressants for them because they have friends they claim are happier since they started taking them. I'm averse in my practice to prescribing such drugs anyway, but especially for seniors. A recent National Institutes of Health study "of 595 patients found that antidepressant use was associated with an increased risk of cognitive decline over 4.5 years among depressed patients without cognitive impairment."[39] Too often, in other words, these drugs are the cause of precisely what the patient is trying to prevent.
- **Seek community:** When I drill down with patients in declining health, a virtual constant is loneliness.

They become recluses, either because the state they're in embarrasses them and they don't want to be seen by others, or because their condition makes getting out and around a challenge that may seem insurmountable.

- **Ask for help:** As many get older, for some reason, they wait for the phone to ring instead of picking it up and dialing themselves. Take the initiative and seek counsel from those inside and outside your family whom you trust.

# THE MOVE NO ONE WANTS TO MAKE

Given a choice, extraordinarily few seniors would leave their home of their own volition to move into an assisted living or nursing home environment, and for good reason. There is no clearer demonstration of an increasing lack of control over our lives than such a move becoming a necessity. I have so many patients who are strong candidates for an assisted living situation who steadfastly oppose even considering it.

People are living longer, and for various reasons, some covered in these pages, they are doing so with increased vigor and passion. But there comes a time for many when their physical and potentially mental declines keep them from effectively functioning independently. They become a burden to themselves and their loved ones, in which case a move into some form of assisted living or skilled nursing situation is warranted.

We need to be honest with ourselves about our particular situation. No one understands any mental and physical decline you're experiencing better than you, and you must be honest with yourself about how best to deal with that. If you can no longer manage routine daily tasks, and any coping mechanisms to aid you in that effort are failing, it is likely time for you to consider a lifestyle change. And just as you must be honest with yourself, you must also be honest with your loved ones when considering alternatives, because there are more out there than you think, and the choices are constantly evolving.

On that subject, if you wait until necessity forces your hand in this kind of decision, it's too late. You need to consider your options earlier rather than later, and the fact is some are far more appealing than others. For example, in-law-style housing renovations or additions make up one of the biggest trends in the construction industry.[40] While not necessarily a permanent solution, this alternative can be the perfect compromise in preserving lifestyle and resources while keeping you close to those you love.

Here are some steps and strategies to ease the transition for you or a loved one for whom you're a primary caregiver.

## PRESCRIPTIONS FOR MAKING THE MOVE NO ONE WANTS TO MAKE

- **Attitude:** Keep an open mind about the alternatives before you honestly assess your situation. If you are considering this kind of change to your lifestyle, chances are you, or someone who is or feels responsible for you, believes the time has come for such a major move. You can't make the clock go backward, so focus on doing what's right for the present into the future.

Try to look at your new lifestyle as a new adventure where the pluses outweigh the minuses.

- **Don't wait until you have to do it:** I have had patients who waited too long to consider their living options for the next phase of their lives. The legendary baseball executive Branch Rickey once said, "It's better to trade a player a year too early than a year too late." The earlier you and your loved ones search for the optimal setting or option for you, the less pressure you will be under, and the more you will be able to mentally prepare for this next stage of your life. Once you find the right living situation, ideally you will look forward to moving in for the strain it takes off you and the burden it lifts from your loved ones.
- **Do your homework:** Research the facilities you're considering by reading the online reviews, and if possible, talk to residents and/or their family members to help educate yourself on the pluses and minuses of your options. Tour the facilities, and trust your gut when you find the one that feels most like your new home even before you move in.
- **Make the space your own:** Decorate your room with familiar photos, keepsakes, and possessions to create a sense of home. You may be leaving the home you've loved, but the more you can create a facsimile of it, the easier your transition will be.
- **Manage your expectations:** You cannot expect your new situation to mirror your old in all ways. This choice is likely being forced on you, so you must not let the perfect become the enemy of the good. So, too,

focus on the positives of your new lifestyle instead of dwelling on the negatives.

- **Communicate needs clearly:** When you sit down with the appropriate parties to help determine your decision, make sure they understand precisely what your needs are and that you understand how they intend to meet them. This is a difficult-enough process without having to repeat it all over again because the choice you made proves to be the wrong one.

# DEALING WITH THE DECLINING HEALTH OF A LOVED ONE

The pressure placed on caregivers for a loved one whose mental and/or physical health is in a state of decline is immense. It can often feel like you're watching someone you love, usually a parent or other close relative, slip away right before your eyes. You can feel helpless in the face of that, and the effects can dominate your life, along with a sense of obligation and responsibility to do everything you can toward that loved one's well-being.

That, though, can become an impossible burden to bear on top of what you're already shouldering. It can be challenging for a spouse, because dealing with the loss of a partner can feel like losing a part of themselves, even *all* of themselves. So when patients come to me who are dealing with this especially painful part of life, my advice to them varies according to their relationship. For the most part, the advice I give a sibling will be different from what I advise a husband or wife, which is different from my advice to a son or daughter.

To cope effectively as a caregiver, it's crucial to prioritize self-care. You *must* not let whatever is ravaging your loved one claim two lives instead of one. I tell my patients cast into this role that they need to set up an early warning system to flash, like a "check engine" light in a car, when they've pushed themselves beyond their limits. The warning signs include:[41]

- If you feel anxious or constantly exhausted
- If you find yourself with no patience or tolerance for other loved ones
- If you have trouble sleeping
- If you have no desire to do what you've always enjoyed
- If you stop exercising, eating right, and generally taking care of yourself
- If you are overcome by sadness that doesn't abate

Each relationship brings its own set of emotional challenges, but I'd like to focus here on general advice that applies to all.

## PRESCRIPTIONS FOR DEALING WITH THE DECLINING HEALTH OF A LOVED ONE

- **Seek support:** You can't do this alone. But if you are forced to manage this burden on your own, you might consider turning to hospice or another form of palliative care. Your instinct is to keep your loved one home and comfortable for as long as possible. There comes a time, though, when that's no longer best for either of you, and you need to rethink everything and know that it's time to give your loved ones over to the care of professionals while you remain an active and supportive presence in their lives.

- **Educate yourself:** You aren't the first person to go through this any more than your loved one is. Hospice counselors can be masterful at advising you on what to expect and how best to cope. You may also have friends or co-workers who've been through what you're going through. Reach out to them as guides so you can better chart the path that lies ahead.
- **Don't walk away:** Nothing is worse than regret over failing to see things through, often as a result of burnout. It's vital to stay strong enough to be there for your loved one, until the time comes to accept you've done everything you can. That's why, against all prevailing instincts, you must moderate your efforts and remember to be as good a caretaker for yourself as you are for your loved one.
- **Practice empathy and patience:** It's natural to resent your loved one for putting you in this position, even hating them at times when the state of your life hits you like a crushing hammer blow. Train yourself to remember that in those times, none of this is their fault or anyone else's. They didn't choose to be in this state, and the best remedy for resentment is to feel their tumult. Even though that may sound counterintuitive to your long-term mental and emotional health, it's a way to preserve the love you feel until the very end and beyond. Patience helps fashion the perspective you need to get through this as whole as you can.
- **Hold fast to your memories:** Nothing can provide more relief to your situation than to hold dear your happy memories. Those memories are like jewels to

cling to and help celebrate the glisten that once lit up your life. Surround yourself with pictures, mementos, and anything that keeps the best version of your loved one at the forefront of your mind, because that is the person you're doing this for.

- **Set new expectations:** Once properly informed, create guidelines to make every day of your loved one's dwindling life as positive and comfortable as possible. Set your expectations low so the smallest victories—a smile, a squeeze of the hand, a softly spoken word—become lights that shine through the darkness.
- **Be realistic:** There's nothing wrong with hope, but expecting or chasing miracles is bad medicine. Set the course and stick to it. Avoid surfing the internet for anything that gives you false hope. While some might call that proclivity chasing a different kind of light, the darkness will only seem more significant when it leads nowhere.
- **Seek professional help:** I have had new patients start psychotherapy during this experience. No two have come to me for the same reasons or have the same needs, but all feel much better just to have a professional, objective party to vent to. These patients will cry in front of me, releasing all the pent-up emotions they tend to repress in front of others.
- **No regrets:** Know in your heart that you are doing everything in your power. Know that you were there until the end while holding on to the essence of the person you're losing at their best. Know that you feel the way you do because of the love they gave you and you have now been able to return in kind when they needed you the most.

# LOSING A LOVED ONE UNEXPECTEDLY

A Chinese philosopher was once asked by a follower to define happiness. He thought for a moment, stroked his chin with a finger, and said, "Grandfather dies, father dies, son dies."

We all dread the ringing of the phone or knock on the door late at night. In fact, the kind of news that can buckle your knees can come at any time.

I've treated any number of patients over the years who've suffered such a loss. Some were already coming to see me, while others began their therapy to help them deal with a loss that had suddenly occurred. It is one thing to deal with grief, but that grief can be magnified several times over when shock is added to the mix. We'd like to think these horrible occurrences only happen to other people because we've insulated ourselves against them, until they're visited upon us. These are the words we push into the deepest recesses of our consciousness to avoid the anxiety that merely considering them can make us contemplate.

I've treated any number of patients who constantly fixate on something terrible happening in their lives, foreseeing something that will likely never happen but, at the same time, cannot be ruled out. I can't tell a patient with complete assurance that they won't face a loved one's tragic car accident, suicide, cancer, stroke, sudden heart attack, COVID case, or school shooting—the list is endless. These things, tragically, happen, and no amount of anxious concern can prepare you when they occur. Nothing can.

Losing a loved one brings profound emotional trauma to family and friends. Someone who once felt solid and permanent in our lives becomes accessible only through memories. Coming to terms with this shift is central to the healing process of grief.

When a loved one dies suddenly and tragically, the loss is compounded by trauma. Trauma, in this sense, is an intensely distressing experience that leaves survivors feeling unsafe and helpless. The term "survivor" is used intentionally because those left behind often feel like they are just that: struggling to survive the aftermath. They must navigate not only the pain of their loss but also the deep emotional wounds caused by the way their loved one died.

In cases of tragic loss, the grieving process can become even more complicated and prolonged by the unanswerable questions surrounding the event. Survivors may grapple with the "why" of the tragedy, searching for meaning in something that often defies explanation. Signs that trauma is present and in need of healing include prolonged shock, guilt over not preventing the tragedy, survivor's guilt, persistent thoughts about the circumstances of the death, vivid imaginings of what may have happened, and intense symptoms of grief that interfere with daily life beyond what might be expected.[42]

Nothing I can say here will relieve the immediate aftermath of shock and dismay. Your loved one is gone, and they're not coming back. So, what should you do to regain some semblance of normalcy and stability in your life? How can you push forward into the future when the present is shrouded by so much despair?

## PRESCRIPTIONS FOR LOSING A LOVED ONE UNEXPECTEDLY

- **Stick to a routine:** Those patients I've had who were stricken by grief in the wake of a sudden loss will often tell me they have trouble finding a reason to get out of bed in the morning. But it's crucial to push yourself to get up and out, resume your routine, and stake as much of a claim to a sense of normalcy as you can manage. Even if you haven't returned to work yet, force yourself to get up at your usual time and go about your day to the best of your ability. The more you wallow in your grief over the sudden loss you've experienced, the more likely it is to consume your life.
- **Be active:** Sitting in your chair or on your couch and staring into space will only worsen your grief and leave you digging into a rut you keep falling back into. Do something physical and positive. You've heard me mention exercise on these pages repeatedly, and you will need to do just that to concentrate on something other than your pain. Every minute of positive distraction

and focus brings you closer to regaining some measure of your happiness.

- **Diet:** This is another theme we've hit on throughout this book, but one that bears repeating. I've had many grief-stricken patients over the years who tell me they've lost their appetite. Sure, I advise them to eat well, but at this point, eating anything is a step in the right direction. Eat meals as close to the same time every day as possible to reestablish a routine and train your mind to look forward and heal.
- **Be strong for others:** I urge patients to be strong for others and become part of their support system. It may sound counterintuitive to do so when your spirits are so down, but a great strategy to lift them is to be there for others who are suffering too. Check in regularly with those who feel the loss as deeply as you do. If you lose a child or partner, find the strength in yourself to be there for your other children or partner. This positive coping mechanism will lend purpose and direction to your life.
- **Be patient with yourself:** There is often no remedy for sudden and tragic loss other than time, as hard as that may be to accept. You want to be as happy as you were before you received that call or answered a late-night knock on the door. But it could take around a year for that to happen, and even then, you need to accept that your definition of happiness will never be the same. Grief over sudden loss spreads a cloud over your life. And, just as you must wait for the literal cloud to pass, so too you need to wait for the figurative one to pass too.

- **Allow others to grieve as they choose:** No one grieves the same way, and what works for you may not work for them. Just as you must be patient with yourself, you must be patient with others, even if you disagree with their approach. I've had patients who visit the grave of the loved one they've lost every day and others who never return to the cemetery at all after the funeral. I've had patients who want to turn the room of a child they've lost into a shrine and patients who want to box up that child's possessions in much shorter order. There is no right way to deal with such a life-changing tragedy. There is only your way.
- **Find a support group or therapist:** Joining such a group puts you in the company of like-minded members of a club no one chose to be a part of but who find a strong support system among those who understand their pain. For some, in-person meetings are most effective, while others gravitate toward such groups on Facebook or websites devoted to survivors like yourself. If such support yields even a single coping mechanism that has worked for someone else, then the effort has been worth it. The members of such a group may also be able to recommend the right psychotherapist if you don't already have a preferred one.
- **Honor the memory of your loved one:** If you came to me, I might ask you to tell me some of the things the loved one you are grieving enjoyed doing the most. I might also recommend using one of those interests to honor their memory. What about organizing a 5k in their honor if they were a runner? What about establishing a scholarship in their name if they were a scholar

or artist? If they loved soccer, what about sponsoring an annual tournament so their memory enriches dozens of others? Those are all examples of things patients of mine have done. The list of possibilities is endless; the labor and passion it takes to pull off something like this can be the best prescription to help you find your new normal. But don't jump into such an effort too quickly. You'll know when it's time.

# COPING WITH POST-TRAUMATIC STRESS DISORDER

We often associate post-traumatic stress disorder, or PTSD, with soldiers returning from combat overseas. But the reality is it can strike anyone who has suffered a profound and unexpected loss. Outside of war, that could be a person losing their business or job, experiencing a financial calamity, losing their home to catastrophe, getting a bad diagnosis, suffering a devastating loss that leads to despair, or enduring the aftermath of even the successful treatment for a disease like cancer. Generally, PTSD is caused by a sudden and dramatic change forced on us by circumstances beyond our control. Unlike grief, though, time alone may not provide remedy or improvement. PTSD can be a devastating psychological condition characterized by a sufferer losing more and more of the light from their world until the darkness is everywhere. Drug addiction, homelessness, and suicide are only a few of the potential by-products of this affliction when left untreated.[43]

The first thing you must do is determine whether you have PTSD, which tends to bring with it several identifiable symptoms that cause an often dramatic shift in your normal behavior and emotions. Let's call this the **"If you"** list:[44]

- If you are plagued by unsettling memories and thoughts
- If you find yourself lashing out and getting angry without reason or provocation
- If you find yourself relying on alcohol or drugs
- If you no longer seek or enjoy the company of friends and loved ones
- If you don't care about your own well-being, leading you to take risks
- If you are no longer interested in things you used to enjoy
- If you are suffering from extreme anxiety

Although we're going to look at some strategies and practices that can relieve the symptoms of PTSD, this is a psychological condition that often requires professional intervention to treat and ultimately resolve. So let's first look at some traditional and innovative approaches to help the patient feel better.

## PRESCRIPTIONS FOR DEALING WITH PTSD

- **Cognitive processing therapy (CPT):** CPT first identifies and then helps the kind of repetitive negative thinking that is roiling a PTSD sufferer's life. That proclivity manifests itself in what experts in the field call "stuck points" that keep the patient from progressing beyond the original causation of the trauma. It helps patients move beyond these stuck points by instilling new cognition patterns that rewire their thought processes. Instead of open-ended, it's usually a twelve-week program to allow a move into another form of therapy in short order if it fails to produce results.[45]

- **Prolonged exposure (PE) therapy:** PE relies more on getting a patient to directly confront the trauma-related memories and causation they may have been avoiding to make progress and move forward with their lives. The specially trained therapist exposes the patient to these triggers in a controlled environment to relieve guilt and the tendency of people living with PTSD to relive the event in question over and over again.[46]
- **Eye movement desensitization and reprocessing (EMDR):** EMDR involves moving your eyes a specific way while you process traumatic memories, the goal being to help put the trauma behind you. Trauma can overwhelm the way the mind processes information, leaving the memory stuck as though the experience is still happening and preventing the sufferer from moving past it. EMDR therapists utilize something called "bilateral dual attention stimulation," basically side-to-side eye movements, to help change the way memories are stored to get past the trauma.[47]
- **Cognitive behavioral therapy (CBT):** The CBT type of psychotherapy aims to help people manage mental health issues by identifying and challenging unhelpful thought patterns and learning practical strategies to change their behaviors. Its primary focus is on the connection between thoughts, feelings, and actions to improve coping mechanisms. Cognitive therapy helps

people learn to replace negative thought patterns with more positive and less harmful ones.[48]

- **Group therapy:** An age-old practice that can still be highly effective for some patients, group therapy is centered on a collection of people sharing thoughts that lift them from the despair of believing it's them against the world. Building empathy for those in the group by members sharing their stories also helps patients build empathy for themselves, helping them understand their suffering better, which is often the first step to relieving it.
- **Prescription-based therapy:** PTSD is one of those psychological afflictions that I would consider a regimen of properly prescribed medications to treat. Since I normally shy away from doing so with my patients, I might well refer the sufferer to a psychiatrist who specializes in PTSD or a psycho-pharmacologist if I arrive at that diagnosis while treating them. Antidepressants, antianxiety medications, atypical antipsychotics, and alpha-1 blockers may be the only thing holding a PTSD sufferer's head above water until they learn how to swim on their own again.

These approaches, though, should not usually be considered as your first line of defense, except in the severest cases of PTSD. Here are simpler, more basic strategies you can practice alone as that initial line to see if some combination makes you feel more like yourself again.

- **Educate yourself:** Understand what trauma is and how it can result in a less pronounced form of PTSD known as "trauma brain," a very real condition that restricts memory and can make carrying out daily tasks difficult. Before you can treat such a condition, you have to acknowledge that it exists and that you are suffering from it.

- **Identify your triggers:** Before you can eliminate the triggers that lead to an episode of anger, withdrawal, or self-destruction, you have to objectively come to grips with what those triggers are. If, for example, a person lost their child in a car accident, an episode might be triggered by hearing the screeching of brakes or the blare of an ambulance's siren. Once you know your triggers, you can mitigate their negative effects on you by training your mind to think of something else, something positive and calming, immediately.
- **Support groups:** PTSD has many causes, but the symptomatic similarities make any sufferer a prime candidate to take comfort that they are not alone. Think of such support groups as "Trauma Anonymous," and joining one can create a sense of community that has a clear notion of what you're going through.
- **Practice proactive relaxation:** This could be medication, yoga, running, exercise, or practicing a more spiritually based martial art like tai chi or aikido. These pursuits focus your thinking inward instead of fixating on the outward thoughts that continue to torment you. In that respect, such practices help rewire the circuitry of your brain in a manner comparable to one of the more professional therapies covered earlier in this section.
- **Activities that make you feel good about yourself:** Hobbies like cooking, model-ship building, furniture

making, car restoration, and coin or stamp collecting help imbue you with a sense of accomplishment and completion that can also serve to retrain the brain by turning its focus away from whatever created the lingering trauma. It could be a new pursuit or something you've long enjoyed but may have drifted away from. There are no wrong answers here. Find what works for you.

- **Get back to a routine:** People often perceive themselves as prisoners of their routines, but those same routines can also provide a cushion for our lives by serving up much-needed consistency we can rely on. Getting into a routine often comes with increased productivity, which provides solace and achievement.
- **Avoid negativity:** That includes triggers like people who annoy you, media reports that make you anxious, or activities you anticipate with dread. Suffering from trauma should grant you permission to stay away from those people, turn off the television, not read the newspaper or social media, and say no to things you don't want to do.

# PART FIVE
# YOUR INTIMATE SELF

*Real intimacy is only possible to the degree that we can be honest about what we are doing and feeling.*

—DR. JOYCE BROTHERS

*A seventy-year-old man who was a regular patient of mine came in for his session smiling more than he had since he lost his wife to cancer several years before.*

*"What's gotten into you?" I asked him.*

*"I met somebody, and I think I'm in love. I never thought I'd feel that way again."*

*The intimate self knows no age, gender, or sexual preference. So, too, intimacy means different things to different people. That definition may or may not include sex, the frequency of which is also up to each individual couple's preference and prerogative. How many times in this book have you heard me say something to the effect that the human psyche is not a one-size-fits-all proposition? The heart knows what the heart wants, and my patient hadn't been looking for a relationship when he met the second woman of his dreams, with whom he shared many of the same interests.*

*He shifted in his chair. "Can you prescribe that pill for me?"*

*"You mean Viagra?"*

*"Or that other one."*

*"Cialis."*

*"Right. You know what they say, Dr. Gilberg, about the spirit being willing but the body, well, not so much."*

*After the woman accepted his marriage proposal, he asked me to officiate at the wedding in my capacity as an ordained rabbi, and I happily agreed.*

*"Why me, though?" I asked him.*

*"I thought you'd tell me I was crazy for falling in love again at my age, but you didn't. Instead, you encouraged me."*

*Men and women at any age in their adult lives deserve love and whatever level of intimacy they choose, however they define both. In my experience, love between two people remains the most positive and powerful force there is. I always encourage my patients when they bring it up, because people have a right to be happy and fulfilled at any age.*

# REMAINING SEXUALLY ACTIVE

Sex is one of the true universal concepts of life. With very few exceptions, it is a prime component of a person's happiness, self-esteem, relationships, and identity for much of their adolescent and adult lives. So it almost sounds simplistic to say that being and/or remaining sexually active remains among the highest priorities in the lives of practically everyone.

The psychological manifestations of sexuality were first raised openly in contemporary times by Sigmund Freud when he discussed the vital role it and intimacy play in our development and our lives. According to a study reported by *The Journal of Sexual Medicine*, "55% of men and 45% of women reported being sexually active, with positive correlations to physical activity like walking, social engagement through club participation, a healthy lifestyle (no tobacco, fewer medications), good mental health, and a positive quality of life; conversely, sexual inactivity was significantly linked to various health issues including cancer, cardiovascular disease, bladder/bowel problems, poor vision, and specific conditions like hearing loss and dementia in men, or skin problems and joint issues in women."[49]

Yet there are some interesting trends to take note of, societal and sociological changes that have altered the paradigm for sexuality. Take this study covering the period ranging from 1991 to 2021:[50]

- Among high school students, 70.7 percent of boys and 69.4 percent of girls have never had sexual intercourse.
- Between 1991 and 2021, the percentage of high schoolers who never engaged in sexual intercourse increased from 45.9 to 70 percent.
- Between 1991 and 2021, the percent of high school females who had never engaged in sexual intercourse increased from 49.2 to 69.4 percent.
- Between 1991 and 2021, the percent of high school males who had never engaged in sexual intercourse increased from 42.6 to 70.7 percent.

These numbers form a stark contrast with the generation at the other end of the spectrum. Indeed, older Americans aged sixty-five and beyond are having more sex, while high schoolers are having less. According to *U.S. News & World Report,* "Forty percent of adults aged 65 to 80 are sexually active, and more than half, 54 percent, say sex is important to their quality of life.... Forty-six percent of 65- to 70-year-olds reported being sexually active, compared to 39 percent of 71- to 75-year-olds and 25 percent of 76- to 80-year-olds."[51]

There are any number of reasons why older adults are enjoying sex longer, and those reasons can be extended to folks in their fifties too. It starts with the availability of safe drugs like Cialis and Viagra, neither of which carries an embarrassing stigma any longer. I've already explained why I don't typically prescribe traditional psychiatric drugs. I do prescribe these, though, and have seen my patients engaging in fulfilling sex lives in numbers that correspond to the statistics quoted above.

Believe it or not, another factor behind older adults enjoying sex longer and better is the prevalence of social media sites geared toward those in this age group. That's right, such apps are not limited to younger adults. Those eligible for Social Security are using the likes of SilverSingles, eHarmony, Match, DateMyAge, and OurTime in increasing numbers, blowing up the myth that this generation missed out on the dot-com era.

That said, adults of any age who maintain active sex lives need to be cognizant of several realities.

## PRESCRIPTIONS FOR YOUR INTIMATE SELF

- **Overall health:** It's not rocket science to conclude that the healthier you are overall, the more, and more often, you will enjoy sex. Diet and exercise, not surprisingly, play a vital role here, as they have frequently throughout this book. Add not smoking, not being overweight, not consuming too much alcohol, and having a strong psychological foundation and you can remain sexually happy and active pretty much indefinitely.
- **Intimacy:** Friends can be intimate and share pretty much everything without having sex. More and more in my patients, I see an evolving relationship dynamic in which friends grow into lovers. That's an excellent prescription for fulfilling sex, because you already enjoy the person's company.

- **Communication:** One of the most positive manifestations of the MeToo movement is that people are less likely to take sex for granted or treat it as an expectation. Men and women are increasingly respectful of each other's wishes and priorities. While I find the so-called consent forms that were popular in colleges for a stretch laughable, both partners must agree on where, when, and how.
- **Social media sites:** As mentioned above, older adults use these in increasing numbers, but younger adults were there long before. There are many such sites, far too many to list here. Advertising lures many younger people to those with the most significant media budgets. Still, in my patients, I've found referrals to be the most successful means of choosing a site to test the dating waters.
- **It's not just the sex...:** I've often said to patients that if sex is the only thing keeping you together, the relationship won't last. I've had many patients over the years who enjoy wonderful, fulfilling relationships that rarely include sex and sometimes not at all. I know of happily married couples who sleep in separate rooms. It's a huge misnomer to equate love and sex. While the former leading to the latter is a prescription for a healthy relationship, the latter leading to the former is a rare occurrence indeed.

# FINDING LOVE AGAIN

Finding love again after being widowed or divorced is the rule, not the exception. According to the Pew Research Center, somewhere around three-quarters of all those who are divorced ultimately marry again. This compares to closer to half of all widowers and widows. Interestingly enough, according to the National Widowers' Organization, 61 percent of men who've lost their wives remarry compared to only 19 percent of women who've lost their husbands.[52] I'm a bit skeptical of such a dramatic split, but not of the general proclivity on its own.

The bottom line is that people rightfully deserve another chance at love and companionship. I married my second wife when I was seventy-two. That was fifteen months after we started dating, and she told me I waited too long.

The example of a patient of mine presents another case study. This patient lost his wife in June, coincidentally at the age of seventy-two. A woman he had known for years, who had been married to his late golf partner, reached out with condolences, and they started dating within a few weeks and were a couple by August before marrying a year or so after that. Some might question if that was too soon or if enough time had passed. I answer them with another question: How much exactly is enough? It's a loaded question because the answer is there are no absolutes, no right or wrongs necessarily. Every individual needs to find what's right for them, in addition to who.

In my patients who lose a partner to death or divorce, there are certain factors I've observed that are relevant here. The example of the patient above supports the first. He ultimately found love again through someone he was already well acquainted with from traveling in the same social circle for many years. He hadn't even seen the woman he'd ultimately remarry since his friend's, her husband's, funeral. But they already knew each other, so their burgeoning relationship smoothed his transition out of grief. His wife had suffered through a long illness, and I've found when that is the case, as opposed to sudden loss, the person is more likely to seek a new relationship faster since they have "pre-grieved" through their months of serving as a caregiver.

In my practice, I've observed that those who've been divorced or widowed and lack a strong existing social connection take considerably longer to find a new partner. These individuals may have already been more isolated and lack the social outlets that allow them to meet people. The larger one's social circle, the more likely they are to either know someone who's also lost their partner or to have friends telling them that there's someone they'd like them to meet. That's why socialization at any age is vital for all of us. Humans aren't wired for isolation or a solitary lifestyle, for the most part.

Let's explore some factors involved in finding love again at any age.

## PRESCRIPTIONS FOR FINDING LOVE AGAIN

- **Timing:** There's no prescription for this. Everyone grieves or recovers differently and must find their own path. I've had many patients who've suffered the loss of their partner ask me over the years, "Doctor, how do I know it's time to move on?" My answer to them is that they'll just know. I urge them not to rush or try to do it on a timetable that worked for someone else. *Patience* is another term I've mentioned frequently, and it applies here yet again.
- **Instincts:** I've found that oftentimes, there's no such thing as being "ready" for a new relationship. The relationship finds you more than the reverse. Someone new or old enters your life and makes you smile, laugh, or enjoy life again. You find chemistry with this person and look forward to seeing them again as soon as you've parted. Maybe there's a follow-up email or phone call. Perhaps the two of you share interests that could stimulate and strengthen the relationship further.
- **Don't rush:** Sometimes the worst way to find the perfect new life partner is to look for one. Let me explain. As humans, we crave companionship. Enjoy dinner, a show, or a movie without any pressure to go further. But you know what? For some people, having someone to spend quality time with dining or traveling is enough. It's right for them. Remember that intimacy and physical attraction lead different people to different places.
- **Feeling good about you:** I've observed people forcing themselves into new relationships without first fully

rebuilding their own lives. We are often with someone for so long that you become a "we" instead of an "I." With that in mind, you need to rebuild the "I" in terms of knowing who you are and how you feel about yourself before you can become a successful "we" again.

- **Support structure:** The more you feel loved and supported outside of your lost relationship, the less likely you are to withdraw. Enjoying the company of people is a strong precursor to finding a person you want to be with. And the support structure around you functions as an emotional bridge to the next stage of your life.
- **Expansion:** You may meet someone with similar interests, like golf or tennis. It could be someone you've met at a casino you frequent or a wine tasting you attend. Continuing to do these things is, of course, vital. But so is a willingness to try something new, or perhaps even do so specifically to meet someone new. I've had patients who've met their new partners on singles cruises and taking flying or scuba diving lessons. It will likely be something you've always wanted to do anyway, which gives you the excuse to do so.
- **Therapy:** This is a time when psychotherapy can be especially beneficial. Sometimes, patients come to me seeking not so much help as permission. And by permitting them to move forward, I'm helping them. Seeing a professional after losing a partner to death or divorce enables you to realize you're not the first and nor are you alone. A psychotherapist can help guide you down a road they have led others along, often by not providing the right answers so much as asking the right questions.

# HEALTHY MIND AND BODY EQUALS EXTENDED SEXUALITY

People enjoy sex later in life because, generally, they stay healthier longer. The intrinsic connection between those two things is as undeniable as it should be obvious. For men, the desired results from a prescription for Cialis or Viagra can only be achieved if they aren't facing other significant health issues that may rule out such drugs in the first place. There is no catch-all formula for having sex late into life beyond this: *Take care of yourself.*

If that was so simple, why aren't more people doing it? Why aren't more people committing to do just that younger in life and ingraining the habit into their lifestyle? Reportedly, on his ninety-second birthday in 1979, the great jazz musician Eubie Blake said, "If I'd known I was going to live so long, I would have taken better care of myself."

Dr. Folasade P. May, a gastroenterologist and associate professor of medicine at UCLA, offers a strategy to address precisely that. "Each year, make a commitment during your birthday month to schedule all your annual health checkups. Schedule them for anytime in the next year before your next birthday. Keeping your health in check requires consistent care. This helps make sure that you get it done."[53]

Taking care of yourself mentally and physically is the surest strategy to extend not only your sexual performance and enjoyment but also the pleasure you take in everything you do. I've had patients who express how miserable they are being on a diet. But they're only on diets because they're thirty pounds overweight. I've had patients who express similar misery over missing the parts of their lives they've lost to age and infirmity, especially sexual drive and performance. Well, there's nothing anyone can do about age, but there's plenty we can all do about infirmity.

And it's never too late. I had a patient who came to me because he was severely depressed over a heart condition that had stolen his sex life from him. He blamed genetics, all the medications he was taking, and a lack of attraction for his partner. He blamed everything except himself. Then, he suffered a minor heart attack, which forced him into a cardiac rehab program. After several months, he lost weight, built stamina, had his medications reduced, and found himself newly attracted to his partner. His depression was as much rooted in his loss of interest in sex as in his inability to perform. These two factors go hand in hand.

However, such dysfunction is not limited to older people. I have had younger patients so busy chasing their futures, putting in fourteen hours a day at law and investment firms, that their success comes at the expense of everything else. They come to me because they want to be happy and deem themselves depressed. It turns out, almost invariably, that their physical and mental health are barely being prioritized. These are thirty- and forty-year-olds walking around in the bodies of sixty- or seventy-year-olds. My prescription for them is to change their lives by changing their priorities.

"Habits like smoking, poor diet, and a sedentary lifestyle can lay the groundwork for heart disease long before the symptoms appear," Nina Agrawal wrote for the Well pages of *The New York Times* in January 2025. These habits "won't kill you the next day, but they may dictate how you live in the last decades of your life," adds Dr. Kyla Lara-Breitinger, a cardiologist and assistant professor of medicine at the Mayo Clinic.[54]

Let's look at a few prescriptions that can best help you maintain the healthy mind and body you'll need to enjoy sex now and long into the future.

## PRESCRIPTIONS FOR STAYING SEXUALLY ACTIVE

- **Strength in routine:** The simplest things can work wonders, like getting up at the same time every morning and going to bed at the same time every night. It's also easier to make exercise a part of your routine when you take a walk or go to the gym at the same time every day. This works especially well for retired people because it provides the discipline they have lost in leaving the workplace.
- **Stress management:** Little can detrimentally affect sexual desire and performance more than stress. Some stress is difficult to control, especially when it involves

a family member struggling financially or personally. I know my patients can't separate themselves from the plights of their children any better than I can, so I urge them to do their best to store different parts of their lives in different compartments. If you can close the door on that compartment after doing everything you can, the stress you feel is less likely to drag you down.

- **Don't over- or self-medicate:** All medications have side effects, and not all are the ones you experience or are mentioned in the voiceover on the television commercials. You'll seldom hear "unable to perform sexually" listed among those, but it happens. The same holds true for alcohol or any drug. I have even noted that patients who initially try Viagra or Cialis often become dependent on them to perform at all.
- **Consult a health-care professional:** If your sexual health, desire, or performance is not what you want it to be or has declined precipitously as of late, see your doctor to discern whether any underlying medical conditions are responsible.
- **Communication:** A good sex life can be a prime component of your relationship, but it should never come to define that relationship. I have found that the better a couple communicates, the more they have sex and the more they enjoy it.
- **Go to sleep:** Another simple prescription that can have a dramatic effect on your well-being in all respects, just as not getting enough sleep can produce an equally dramatic opposite effect by "increasing your stress hormones, promoting inflammation that can lead to plaque buildup in the arteries. It can disrupt your

circadian rhythm and impair your metabolism."[55] If you want to continue having sex late into life, make sure you use the bed for sleeping too!

- **The erotic thread:** That phrase was coined by Dr. Ian Kerner, PhD, LMFT, a psychotherapist and sex therapist. "Too many couples get hung up on sex," he explains, "either the sex they're having or the sex they're not having. I like to focus on what I call the 'erotic thread,' which is the space in between sexual events. A tease, a squeeze, a peek, a poke, a flirtatious text, a melt-into-each-other embrace—little erotic charges that bring some heat into our daily lives and maintain a sense of sexual playfulness."[56]

# BEING LGBTQ+

According to NPR, Americans who identify as lesbian, gay, bisexual, transgender, or queer (LGBTQ) have doubled in roughly the past decade from 3.5 percent of adults in 2012 to 7.6 percent in 2023.[57] The same survey conducted by Gallup found that the number of LGBTQ individuals has consistently increased over each of those interim years.

As for younger adults, NBC News recently reported a significantly higher percentage of Gen Z members (born between 1997 and 2012) identify as LGBTQ, fully one-quarter or slightly more than three times the overall average noted above.[58]

"Concerning LGBTQ identity, it's very clear that Gen Z adults look different than older Americans," noted Melissa Deckman, chief executive at the Public Religion Research Institute.[59]

I'm not interested in rehashing battles over the relative merits of statistics and which studies out there may be outliers. The numbers speak for themselves and suggest the undeniable reality that increasing numbers of Americans are openly referring to themselves as either gay, bisexual, lesbian, transgender, or queer. Notice I said "openly," because it is quite possible the actual number hasn't varied or increased so much as the willingness of LGBTQ Americans to express their sexuality publicly.

Who can blame them? Listening to the targeting of transgender youth and adults over the course of the 2024 presidential campaign, you might have thought this oppressed extreme minority of the population was responsible for all of the country's problems. Officials in Huntington Beach, California, for example, have pushed through a new law that requires the likes of teachers, librarians, and others in the city's employ to inform parents if they learn their kids are transgender or gay. "No one has more at stake in the future of a child than that of the parent of that child. The children are not property of the state. The children are under the parent's guidance," said local Councilmember Natalie Moser, commenting on the egregious nature of such overreach and blatant victimization of a community ill-equipped to fight back.[60]

What if you are one of those LGBTQ Americans, whether or not you're public about it? Unfortunately, it means you may find yourself facing very real challenges not faced by straight people that can unfairly and adversely affect aspects of your life. As soon as you identify yourself as LGBTQ, in adolescence or even younger, you may not gain acceptance even among the people you hold most dear, family and friends who unfortunately cannot accept you for who you are and may even ostracize you. Outside of the home, meanwhile, you may find yourself, for one, confronting discrimination in the workplace whereby you are paid less than your straight counterparts and passed over when opportunities for promotion arise, along with a higher unemployment rate than the rest of the population. LGBTQ adults also face discrimination in health care and are much more likely to report negative experiences with the system as a whole. Then, undeniably, there is the harassment that the same adults continue to face in numbers far larger than their straight peers. According to the UCLA School of Law's Williams Institute, "47% of LGBTQ workers have experienced discrimination or harassment at work at some point in their lives," whereas only "12 percent who aren't out have experienced workplace discrimination."[61]

That puts immense pressure on an LGBTQ person's mental, physical, and emotional health. Not surprisingly, their rates of attempted suicide are between three and six times higher than their heterosexual peers.[62] And the disparities among younger people who identify as LGBTQ are even more staggering. According to a 2023 study by the Trevor Project, as reported by ABC News, "41% of LGBTQ young people seriously considered attempting suicide in the past year." Directly related to that is the fact that the same study found "56% of LGBTQ young people who wanted mental health care in the past year were not able to get it."[63]

The shocking disparity indicated in these reports bears mention since that is what as much as 10 percent of the country's population is facing. If you're part of that 10 percent and want to know how to avoid becoming a statistic yourself, you've come to the right place.

Let's look at some ways those who identify as LGBTQ can deal with the irrational pressure society seems bent on placing on them.

## PRESCRIPTIONS FOR THOSE WHO ARE LGBTQ+

- **Find strength in the community:** The LGBTQ community has never been stronger, more supportive, or better organized. I am not referring necessarily to political activism so much as social support, by which I mean settings where you can gather with like-minded individuals who share your values and are bonded by shared experience. This has the tangential effect of providing you with a social network that offers opportunities to meet others.
- **Give back:** Nothing can make you feel better than helping others in any situation, but that is especially true in the LGBTQ community. As the statistics we quoted earlier indicated, LGBTQ youth are in desperate need of adult role models and mentors who can help them negotiate the often fraught path ahead. Helping them walk that path will help you reconcile the struggles you faced at that age and perhaps never fully emerged from. You will feel better yourself by making someone else feel better about themselves.
- **Control:** The old US Army catchphrase, "Be all you can be," applies here as well because you definitively control how you look, act, and feel. Because of the pressures being LGBTQ can place on your mental health, it's even more essential to safeguard your physical health through diet and exercise. And the better you do at that, the more your self-esteem will rise, minimizing the effects the actions and words of haters have on you.

- **Mental health resources:** This is another area where some form of therapy or counseling can prove very beneficial. If psychotherapy isn't for you, you may want to try a support group or group therapy. There is also therapy that relies on more Outward Bound–type activities that test your physical limitations in the company of others facing comparable challenges to strengthen your mental and emotional health. You need to find what works best for you, even if it takes a bit of trial and error. But never be afraid to ask for help.
- **Affirmative therapy:** Practiced by a specialist in this particular field, affirmative therapy aims to strengthen a patient's acceptance of their identity by celebrating it. The vast majority of the patients I've seen over the years come to me due to experiences or conditions that have negatively affected their lives. But the root cause of emotional turmoil for the LGBTQ community lies in identity, not experience. Affirmative therapy provides a safe space in which the patient is under no pressure to be anyone but themselves as they work through the issues, challenging their emotional health by setting clear and modest goals that help them embrace the very identities they have viewed as the root of their problems.[64]

# HAVING A CHILD OR GRANDCHILD WHO IS LGBTQ+

Inevitably, as the LGBTQ population rises among younger people, it becomes more likely you will have a child or grandchild who comes out. I do not believe sexuality is any more of a conscious thought than hair or eye color. You can dye your hair or wear colored contact lenses, but there's no such convenient mechanism for a person to change the sexuality they were born with. The best thing you can do for your child's or grandchild's mental health is to accept them for what they are and encourage them to do the same for themselves.

I will concede this has proved to be a tumultuous issue for my patients over the years. Initially, they have expressed some combination of shock, dismay, resentment, blame, and denial—in short, how the news they've received affects them. Inevitably, I turn the conversation back to their child and grandchild.

*What else is different about them?*

*Are they the same person as they were the day before you got the news, besides this one exception?*

*I understand how you feel. Now tell me how* they *feel?*

Almost invariably, in answering those questions, the parent or grandparent will start to come around to the fact that their child's or grandchild's sexuality belongs to them and them alone and that their happiness in being who they were born to be rises above all other concerns. The positive news is over my many years of practice, there has been an appreciable trend toward acceptance and away from the stigma. A 2019 AARP survey found that 88 percent of grandparents said they would accept a grandchild who came out to them as LGBTQ.[65]

Too often still, though, my patients are looking for someone to blame. At times, they look toward the child or grandchild themselves for making a choice with which they strongly disagree. I remind them that a person's sexuality is determined at birth and not the result of a conscious decision on their part. I urge them to celebrate and support their child's or grandchild's decision to finally accept their true identity.

"Do you want them to be happy?" I ask. The answer is always yes. I tell them all people have a right to be happy, and living outside their own identity impeded that for their child or grandchild. They were pretending to be someone they were not, wearing a costume every day while their inner conflict and turmoil threatened to ruin their lives. I urge my patients to do everything they can to love and support the child or grandchild now, because this is when they need that love and support more than ever. By coming out, they are giving notice that they are finally coming to accept themselves, and it would be an extreme disservice not to accept them in kind.

A patient may ask me, "Even if I'm slow in coming around, what should I do?" Here are some of the steps I might advise them to take.

## PRESCRIPTIONS FOR HAVING AN LGBTQ CHILD OR GRANDCHILD

- **Show your love:** A kiss or even a hug can do more than words. For some, this comes naturally. For others, long-held beliefs may get in the way of being able to respond positively and supportively. Keep this in mind, though: No matter how difficult learning about your child's sexual orientation or gender identity can be for you, it was likely even more difficult for them to finally inform you of their true sexual identity. In another sense, them telling you the truth is the ultimate act of love, and that's the way it should be returned, no matter what deep-seated opinions may be getting in the way.
- **Get past yourself:** This isn't about you. It's not your life. There have been times when a patient's response to a child or grandchild coming out is so obstinate and demeaning, I ask them, "Don't you think it's selfish of you to feel that way?" Over time, even some of my most ardent patients in that regard will come around. As for the ones who can't, I urge them not to draw a line in the sand that could potentially devastate or even end the relationship, which regrettably does happen. I encourage those with that mindset to observe the responses of others in the family, and if those responses are markedly different, I ask them to examine what is

behind their stubbornness when someone they love needs them the most.

- **Support:** Your job as a parent or grandparent is to support, not judge. When I drill down into what's happening, several patients have said something to the effect of, "Now I won't be able to have grandchildren." First off, that's not true and represents being misinformed. Support means informing yourself as best you can about how little this changes the opportunity for your child or grandchild to build a warm and loving family for themselves. According to a study reported by the Faulkner Law Group, the divorce rate for straight couples stands at 46 percent compared to only 17 percent for gay couples.[66] Additionally, increasing numbers of gay couples are having children, either through adoption or a surrogate—somewhere between 15 to 20 percent despite the challenges presented.
- **Join the club:** Earlier in this chapter, we presented statistics that the gay population of the United States hovers somewhere around 10 percent, which means you're now a member of a club that's much larger than you may have thought. And there are ample support groups for parents and grandparents of gay kids sponsored by the likes of PFLAG (Parents, Families, and Friends of Lesbians and Gays). I recommend checking into this group.
- **Encourage:** In many, if not most, cases, the child or grandchild was aware of their sexual identity and was likely acting on it long before they had this conversation with you. It may have taken years for them to work up the courage to finally tell you the truth about who they

are. I tell my patients what their child or grandchild needs at that moment more than anything is encouragement. They need to know you're there for them as much as you were before this conversation started. The first question you should ask is, "How can I help?" If a boyfriend or girlfriend is already in their lives, ask when you can meet them. Often, that person's family may not have been as supportive as you, and there is no better way to show your love for your child or grandchild than to be supportive of their partner as well.

- **Have their backs:** We cited a study earlier that indicated nearly 50 percent of LGBTQ individuals report facing some form of workplace discrimination or general harassment in the preceding year.[67] My point is that your child or grandchild is already facing multiple challenges outside the family. The last thing they need is a family that adds to those challenges. Ask yourself how you would have reacted to them being bullied or abused for an entirely different reason. Your response in their support should be even more demonstrative, because they need you in their corner now more than ever.

# PART SIX
## FAMILIES

*Call it a clan, call it a network, call it a tribe, call it a family: whatever you call it, whoever you are, you need one.*

—JANE HOWARD

*A woman I hadn't seen in a while booked several sessions concerning the anxiety she was feeling over her eighteen-year-old daughter heading off to college.*

*"I remember what it was like when I left her alone as a baby. I couldn't think of anything but her the whole time my husband and I were out. We left without even finishing our anniversary dinner, and that's how I'm feeling again about her getting ready to move a thousand miles away."*

*"Tell me about your daughter."*

*The woman gushed for several minutes, not once tearing up as she reviewed her daughter's accomplishments.*

*"You think her success, all she's achieved, was random?"*

*"She's an incredible girl."*

*"Maybe because you empowered her. Maybe because you gave her everything she needed to become this incredible young woman."*

*The more we talked through the ensuing sessions, the less anxious and more grateful she became, thankful for having raised such a wonderful daughter whose work ethic had gotten her into a top school and whose confidence allowed her to venture far away from home. I told my patient there was nothing wrong with being sad over missing her daughter, but at the same time, she should celebrate the vital part she played in her development.*

# THE FAMILY UNIT

Today, the family dynamic has been redefined to include queer couples with or without children, single-parent households, blended families, adult children returning to the roost, and what I'll call ADU (accessory dwelling unit) families. I've had patients from all five of these, and I can tell you that the seven factors needed to maintain a happy, cohesive family unit equally apply to each. With each, though, there are distinct and challenging dynamics at work.

The family unit is not a cookie-cutter proposition, far from it. Family is what you mold from scratch, what you create for yourself. The traditional family, for example, consisting of parents of the opposite sex parenting children they've had together, has been around the longest and remains the most prevalent. According to recent US Census data, approximately 71 percent of children in the United States are raised in two-parent families.[68]

Anecdotally anyway, we can't assume that the traditional two-parent family unit is a recipe for surefire stability. Just look at the number of perpetrators of mass school shootings who were raised in that environment. Successful family units should not be stereotyped, because we don't know what's happening behind those drawn drapes. That said, let's move on to those seven ingredients to make a happy family.

## PRESCRIPTIONS FOR A HAPPY FAMILY

- **Communication:** Children should know what is expected of them in the household. I've found in my practice that nothing is more important in this regard than children being free to share anything with their parents, the bad and the good. A poor test score, a speeding ticket, an altercation in school, a problem with a teacher—the list is endless. But the reverse must also be true. In families that work best, the parents aren't afraid to share their experiences and opinions with their children as well. That creates trust, and nothing pulls a family down more than when a parent doesn't trust a child or vice versa, just as nothing is more destructive in a family than lying.
- **Shared experience:** So many of our most cherished childhood memories are culled from family trips, going out to dinner or the movies, and vacations where the different environment inspires a new way of looking at each other. No relationship is static, and shared experiences encourage the parent-child relationship to evolve, grow, and thus thrive.
- **Tradition:** Virtually all families have birthdays, holidays, and other traditions that are as reliable and regular as flipping one month to another on a calendar. Traditions provide anchors for both adults and children,

something to hold on to in good and bad times. When good, we celebrate. When bad, we find ourselves putting our problems in context and weighing them against the whole of our lives.

- **Adaptability:** Change happens for any number of reasons. The better a family can adapt to a move that's either forced or chosen helps determine how well they'll be able to maintain their happiness. In my practice, I've found empowering children to have a voice and a seat at the table makes them more adaptable when change comes. It's not just informing them; it's having the ability to pose a question that begins with, "What do you think about..." On the other hand, when the change is seen as forced on them without proper acknowledgment, it becomes much harder for them to accept that change and adapt.
- **Conflict:** Conflict is inevitable. How long it lingers and how well it's resolved will determine whether it becomes a learning experience or an enduring plague on the relationship. I'm not a child psychiatrist, so my knowledge is limited to their parents. And I can't tell you how many of my patients have been roiled by something blown out of proportion over the years. When it comes to conflict, the number one rule must be to keep everything in perspective and never let your child become the adult in the room by your overreacting or lashing out.
- **Support:** As parents (and grandparents), we are wired to support our kids through thick and thin, to stand up for them and have their back, and to love them without any hesitation. As parents, the last thing we

ever want to do is let our kids down. I've had patients thrown into emotional disarray over a turn in finances not enabling them to buy the right gift, continue to pay for college, help buy a car, and so many others. The thing is, I tell them, support cuts both ways. The stronger the relationships you've forged with your kids, the more likely they will understand the situation and stand by your side instead of pulling away. Support, in other words, must be given as well as gotten.

- **Respect:** Respect is something else that should be reciprocal. When patients bemoan their child doesn't respect them, my first questions are, "Do you respect them?" and "Do you respect their decisions instead of wanting them to fit into a premade mold of your creation?" If they choose not to go to college immediately or attend a trade school instead, you must respect that. If they decide to pursue theater or dance instead of sports, you need to respect that. If they come out to you as gay, you need to respect that. Respect and acceptance are not interchangeable, but they are intrinsically connected. And the more you respect your child, the more likely you are to accept their decisions and choices.

# QUEER COUPLES

According to the Williams Institute, 18 percent of LGBTQ adults are parenting children, around five million kids in total.[69] That said, queer couples raising children often face distinct challenges that have brought either a partner or the couple to my office for psychotherapy. They talk about the social stigmas they face. Even the most liberal and welcoming of communities aren't universal in their acceptance of families that are "different" by their very definition. But that dynamic pales in comparison with the myriad of legal issues regarding adoption and surrogacy, not to mention the fear that a changing political climate will ultimately render their entire marriage null and void.

Other queer couples have come to me over the everyday challenges they face in, first, explaining their relationship to their child or children and, second, helping the child or children deal with the ostracism and bullying they may face at school. Unfortunately, kids tend to think in very one-dimensional terms. If Tommy or Tammy's parents are gay, then Tommy or Tammy must be gay too. And in our country, despite the strides made in rectifying both legal and social norms, gay-coupled families still stand out and tend to be treated differently. That's despite the fact research shows that children raised by same-sex parents develop just as well as those raised by heterosexual parents.[70]

## PRESCRIPTIONS FOR QUEER MARRIAGES AND FAMILIES

- **Build a social network:** No matter where you live, you need to establish a strong support system of like-minded, or at least open-minded, individuals. This is your buffer zone, insulation between a normal home life and one that is constantly roiled by your children being ostracized and bullied. Where do the children of those in your circle attend school? What schools have the strongest antidiscrimination policies, most notably zero tolerance when it comes to discrimination of any kind? What social or volunteer efforts can you sign up for that will help ingratiate you with the community for who you are?
- **Early identification:** The earlier your children accept and embrace who you and they are, the more normal it will become for them as they grow into their formative and adolescent years. Suppose they begin to demonstrate signs of stress over dealing with having two parents of the same gender once coming of age. In that case, you may want to consider more formal support groups or even family psychotherapy with a specialist in this field. I have been amazed at the results of early psychiatric intervention in childhood for, if nothing else, giving the child an adult they trust and

with whom they can share their innermost feelings and struggles.

- **A changing landscape:** Children of queer couples face emerging and shifting challenges as they move through grade school, as do children of straight couples. The difference with children of gay couples is this added dynamic they face in carving out their identity. That makes it crucial to accept that even if you do everything right, challenges will likely arise you didn't necessarily plan for or anticipate. That's why it's vital to maintain open communication channels to prevent a problem from festering into a crisis. Something like that needs to be dealt with today, not tomorrow.
- **Sense of self:** The more your child develops their own identity, the happier and more secure they will be. Organized activities of any kind, especially group-oriented ones, can be especially beneficial here, because they encourage your child to develop a strong social circle that will grow with them as they age into young adulthood with the same friendships they've enjoyed since they were as young as five or six years old.
- **Home as the constant:** Even more so than straight couples, queer couples need to maintain a stable home. Their children need to feel this is a safe space they can retreat to, no matter how much they may be struggling with ridicule, ostracism, and even abuse. In a class of fifteen, it only takes one to make another child's life miserable, and it is regrettably impossible for adults to always intervene. Living in a home they can retreat to behind figurative moats and gates becomes their solace, and it's your responsibility to create that space for your children.

# THE SINGLE PARENT

According to the Pew Research Center, a quarter of all children in the United States are being raised in single-parent environments. And, interestingly enough, the US has the highest rate of kids growing up in single-parent households of any developed country in the world.[71]

On their own, those numbers are not entirely surprising, but let's dig a little deeper. Single-parent homes must contend with issues unique to that living environment. Except for cases of adoption or surrogacy by an individual adult, the origins of single-parent homes lie in divorce, or in the other parent having passed away or abandoned their family. In all these scenarios, the kids left to be raised by single parents may well have suffered some degree of discomfort in their lives at best or have been traumatized at worst. The Annie E. Casey Foundation, an organization devoted to the welfare of all children, has found that "while most children in single-parent households grow up to be well-adjusted adults, kids from single-parent families may be more likely to face emotional and behavioral health challenges—like engaging in high-risk behaviors—when compared to peers raised by married parents."[72]

That said, no research suggests that children raised in a household without a mother or father present are at an inherent disadvantage. And most single-parent households are successful, even thriving, in numbers comparable to two-parent households, largely because of the following practices.

## PRESCRIPTIONS FOR SINGLE-PARENT HOUSEHOLDS

- **Prioritize your child or children:** This is the best strategy to ensure a successful and thriving home. Unfortunately, that may mean putting your own career ambitions on hold. You won't be able to travel very much or work long hours at the office past the child's meal or bedtime. Child care and babysitters can only go so far effectively.
- **Finding a new partner:** In my practice, I have found that single-parent patients can often struggle in relationships with other single parents and seem to fare much better in relationships where the other person has no kids or kids who have grown and are on their own. Working both sets of kids into the relationship, particularly at the outset, can be challenging. Alternatively, when only one of the potential partners has a child, it's much easier to involve the child without the messy dynamics of needing to build multiple bonds, not to mention the dynamics between the children themselves.
- **Establish a routine:** That applies to you as well as your child or children, not just to them. Home environments

where the child and parent enjoy breakfast and dinner together are more likely to foster success, even to the point of being associated with lower levels of depression as well as substance abuse.[73] You need to build your schedule around your child so you can attend the games, concerts, plays, or other activities in which they participate. On occasions when you can't be there, your absence is magnified by the fact that often *both* parents for the rest of the kids are there to root their child on.

- **Take care of yourself:** You're no good for your child if you don't take care of yourself. If you can't get to the gym at all or as much anymore, invest in a piece of home workout equipment. Better yet, build into your exercise routine activities you can do with your child or children. Maybe kicking around a soccer ball, shooting baskets, playing catch with a football, hiking, or jogging. Not only are you taking care of yourself, but you're doing so in what passes as quality time.
- **Seek support:** There are books out there that may help, along with support groups that can double as social situations where you might meet someone with whom you already have a great deal in common. Psychotherapy also works for some, especially because it provides you with a safe space to vent to keep you from holding your frustrations and anxiety bottled up inside.
- **Role models:** A grandmother or grandfather can be vital for at least somewhat filling the gap of not having a mother or father in the home. If you're dating someone, even a fellow single parent, be leery of casting them in this role too soon. I've had patients come to me over the years who wanted to break things off with

their new boyfriend or girlfriend but couldn't because they had developed a strong relationship with the other person's child. Patients ask me how they know when to bring their new love interest into their child's lives. My answer, almost invariably, is simple: You'll know.

- **Community:** We've all heard the phrase it takes a village to raise a child. Let's tweak that to say it takes building a community to raise a child in a single-parent household. That would be friends and relatives whom you should strive to make an indelible part of your child's life and yours. Community, of course, is vital in traditional two-parent households as well. Still, it's more important here because it fosters a support system for the child outside of you, which can only increase their sense of well-being and security.

# BLENDED FAMILIES

A blended family is one where both partners have children from their previous lives sharing the home with them. According to the US Census Bureau, around 16 percent of children in the United States live in blended families, which means approximately 40 percent of families with children fall under the blended definition, especially when it's expanded to only one partner having a child from a previous relationship instead of both.[74]

My kids grew up with *The Brady Bunch*, a television show that featured the ultimate blended family, the father's three boys being blended with the mother's three girls. This being television, the show seldom, if ever, strayed into the challenges blended families face in reality. In my years of practice, I've learned that no two blended families are the same. Each comes with its own set of dynamics that can start with age differences. Toddler or early school-age children don't always blend well with children of high school age. It's easy for older kids, who may resent such a major change to their lives in the first place, to resent it even more when they are pressured to spend time with kids ten years their junior who don't necessarily have an off switch. That is not to say blended families with kids of the same general age don't come with their share of potential challenges due to competition and conflict, particularly among teenagers.

Fortunately, I've observed enough successful blended families in my practice over the years to have an informed concept of what made them that way.

## PRESCRIPTIONS FOR BLENDED FAMILIES

- **Consistent messaging:** It helps when the relationship partners enjoy a similar parenting style. However, when those styles don't mesh, creating two sets of expectations and rules laid uneasily over each other, the result can be incessant strife and conflict that fosters resentment on another level. The parents must be on the same page for a blended family to maximize its chances for a great life together. Inconsistent messaging allows the children on either side to pit one parent against another, creating division. When patients contemplate embarking on the path of a blended family, I strongly recommend they seek counseling from a specialist in family therapy to work all this out in advance to preempt the divisiveness that may result otherwise.
- **Communication:** Both partners need to communicate effectively with the children of the other. Don't wait until you're living together under one roof to get to know your new partner's children. That process should be undertaken on both sides before the blending so a comfort zone exists, fostering open channels of communication as soon as the families are blended.

- **Dealing with grief and depression:** Virtually all the time, a blended family emerges out of either divorce or the death of a spouse. So, even if substantial time has passed, it is natural to expect periods where children will revisit the trauma of their loss or separation from their other parent. This is a time when communication is more important than anything else, knowing what to say as well as what not to say or say nothing at all, especially since a typical response to such trauma is to lash out at the substitute parent. Remember, this is not your doing, and the more supportive you can be, the more likely the blended family will emerge unscathed from the experience. If it's your partner's child, follow their lead in how to best approach and deal with the situation.
- **Patience:** If everything goes according to plan, you will spend the rest of your life with your new partner and their children. Things might not, probably won't, click overnight. Don't overreact or over expect. Don't get frustrated when your goodwill overtures are met with resistance or antagonism. Remember that these are children you are dealing with, and it is your responsibility to be the adult in the room, which means being patient.
- **Flexibility and resilience:** A blended family may not be for you if you expect everything to be exactly as you want it. A successful blending requires you to bend your will to the realities around you and the emerging needs of your children, your partner's children, and your partner themselves. In my experience, when blended families don't work, the blame can be laid on a failure or inability to be flexible enough to empower

the new kids in your life so they can better accept you into their lives.

- **New experiences and traditions:** Traveling somewhere neither family has been before can prove an excellent experience for blended families since it represents making brand-new memories instead of evoking comparisons with old ones. It's okay to bond over experiences the new kids in your life are comfortable with, because that will bring you closer to them. Building an identity of its own not based on experiences of one part of the whole brings the new family unit closer together. When the holidays and birthdays come around, celebrating in a new and different way will evoke only happy memories of something comparable, not an experience that's measured against what came before. That said, if there is a venue both halves of the blended family love visiting, like Disney World, that would make a great choice too.
- **Don't forget yourself:** Self-care has been a recurring theme of this book because only if you take care of yourself can you properly take care of the people most important to you. You may want to make this a bonding exercise by engaging with one or more of the new kids in your life who share your healthy interests, such as running, or even less healthy ones, like a favorite TV show. There is no better prescription for the success of a blended family than finding, or forging, common ground by experiencing positive activities together.

# AGING PARENTS AND ACCESSORY DWELLING UNIT (ADU) FAMILIES

As the Baby Boomer generation ages, their offspring are forced to confront a problem that often lacks a viable solution. There aren't a lot of options to pursue when an aging parent or couple can no longer safely and competently take care of themselves. Home health care is prohibitively expensive, especially as the hours increase with the aging person's or couple's needs. And both assisted living and skilled nursing environments are financially onerous as well. The aging person or couple faces the loss of all or most of the resources they've worked to accumulate to ensure effective care in a supportive environment they don't want to be in. Add to that the challenges posed by filling the demands of physical and mental decline, and the roles end up being reversed, with the children placed in the role of being responsible for the needs of their aging parents.

A patient told me not too long ago about going to the drugstore to buy diapers for their infant in one aisle and diapers for their father in the next aisle over. They were trying to be funny but neither of us laughed, because that went to the heart of this patient's challenge.

In large part in response to that challenge, the development of new living environments has become a big trend as of late, with the construction of both in-law apartments and ADUs (accessory dwelling units), which are tiny homes constructed mainly in the rear of an existing property. Zoning laws are being changed to accommodate this increasingly popular trend, which is typically far less expensive than any form of long-term care. Anecdotal studies indicate that elderly parents who move in with their children fare much better than those who move to a facility. In fact, "One out of every four caregivers lives with the elderly or disabled loved one he or she cares for."[75]

With that in mind, let's consider some strategies for this track.

## PRESCRIPTIONS FOR DEALING WITH AGING PARENTS

- **Act early:** If you wait until you have to build an ADU or in-law apartment, it may already be too late. This takes serious and meticulous planning for the next stage of your parents' or parent's life, which will help define your next stage. From a financial standpoint, though, renovating a home or constructing an accessory dwelling is likely to bear a far more reasonable cost than long-term care. Remember, though, this may prove only a stopgap. You are not changing the inevitable so much as postponing it, in all likelihood.

- **Mindset:** Bringing your elderly parent into your space is going to change your life, especially if their decline accelerates. Don't try to fool yourself into believing things will go on like they always have, not when you've accepted responsibility for caring for an aging adult who may no longer be able to take care of themselves fully. Look at the time you've been granted as a means to get to know your parent(s) in a way that brings you back to your childhood and encourages your children to build even closer relationships with their grandparent(s).
- **Engagement:** The more you and your family make your new resident feel at home, the more comfortable they will be and the more likely they will flourish in their new environment. Remember that this move was likely forced on you, and it's just as hard, if not harder, on them as it is on you. Also, keep in mind that your partner is to be celebrated for standing by your side and accepting the new responsibility thrust upon both of you.
- **Have a plan:** This especially refers to finances. Should the time eventually come when the move to a long-term care facility is warranted, be aware of what your parent(s)' finances allow and how long it will likely last. Be cognizant of further decline so you will be able to make the necessary adjustments when either or both mental and physical capabilities wane. You can take steps to prolong your parent(s) stay with you for as long as possible, but you must always be prepared to face the inevitable.

- **Patience:** There's that term again, and for good reason. This isn't going to be easy on anyone. You and your family have made this choice because it was the best option, and it will take time for both you and your parent(s) to adapt to the new environment and new reality. In many cases, one of those children may have given up their own space to make room for Grandma or Grandpa. Always keep in mind how difficult this change is for them, especially in the initial stages.
- **Seek resources:** Is there a senior center in your area that offers activities and social interaction opportunities? If your parent is experiencing cognitive decline, can you utilize an adult day-care center to take some of the strain off you? This is another time when psychotherapy may be warranted, at which point the therapist can help you drill down to the heart of your feelings so that you can better cope with them. Family therapy may help as well.
- **Pace yourself:** Emotionally spent, you're no good to anyone, including yourself. Burnout may lead you to lash out and hold it against your parent, who cannot control the decline that has created the necessity you're facing. Managing realistic expectations for yourself is the best prescription for not damaging your relationship with your partner and/or your children. Trying to do too much is the surest way to ensure you don't do anything as well as you're capable of.

# PARENTING ADULT CHILDREN

Along with the ADUs we covered in the last section, another growing trend among families is adult children moving back in, often into the same space in which they grew up. According to the Pew Research Center, as reported in *USA Today* in December 2021, a staggering 52 percent of adults aged eighteen to twenty-nine lived with their parents.[76] The study cited financial needs as the primary stimulus for a growing trend that contradicts young people's desire to flee the nest. That's no wonder, given the staggering amount of student loan debt many young people amass while in college and/or graduate school, which makes paying rent a difficult, if not impossible, proposition, never mind buying a home because of the debt load they're already carrying.

In the wake of the COVID pandemic, rental costs have soared to the point where finding an affordable apartment can be impossible. Inflation has gone through the roof. The job market has undergone a sea change. These are incredibly challenging times for those starting out and even more challenging for those occupying a low rung on their company's ladder.

Most families will welcome their children back into their midst. Robert Frost once wrote, "Home is the place, that when you go there, they have to take you in." And that's generally the way it is. The vast majority of parents, no matter how reluctant, will willingly open their doors as a way station while their child figures out what happens next. In fact, according to the 2021 census, nearly five million adult children were living with their parents.[77] However, a fair percentage of these returned to a home different from the one they had left because they might find themselves with a new stepmother or stepfather. This adds a new dynamic to the situation and could jeopardize the couple's and parent's relationship with their child if the predicament is not appropriately handled.

There are also instances where an adult child moves back in with their parents because of a health issue. I've had patients, for example, who've told me about their adult child's substance-abuse problem, forcing them to stage an intervention and bring them home to provide a stable environment where they can recover. There are also situations where the adult children have either never gotten their lives together or done so in a destructive manner. Thanks to situations like that, a whole new way of parenting has emerged where the parent(s) take on the same responsibilities they did during their child's grade school years, enforcing discipline and providing order and regimen to their lives.

Whatever has made your adult child return to the nest, there are steps you can take to make the experience as smooth and positive as possible.

## PRESCRIPTIONS FOR PARENTING ADULT CHILDREN

- **Clear expectations:** Do you expect them to contribute financially? Is their return home open-ended, or will you give them a deadline? Do you expect them to take on any responsibilities while living under your roof again? These questions and others need to be answered before their return so they know exactly what is expected of them, including a long-term plan. Forewarned, as the saying goes, is forearmed.
- **Support:** Your adult child is almost surely moving back only after exhausting all other options. It isn't easy for them to do that, much less concede the necessity of the move to you. So this is not the time to criticize or ridicule them or to say some version of "I told you so." This is when they need you to have their backs while they figure out where they go from here to find a sustainable living situation.
- **Discipline:** If they have moved back in because they are out of work, searching for their next position should be part and parcel of the arrangement. They need to know this is what you expect of them in return for that, and they are welcome to stay as long as they continue searching for their next landing spot. Letting them sit around all day, wallowing or playing video games, is not the answer. You may want to encourage them to go back to school or take some online classes in a new discipline they're pursuing. Anything to make sure they don't get too comfortable under your roof, while

fostering a sense of dignity in them. They need to be as productive as possible for everyone's sake.

- **Preparation:** Such a lifestyle change may not be easy for parents or the adult child, so all concerned need to prepare themselves for what's coming openly and honestly. This is especially true if younger siblings are also living at home. The delicate balance of their adolescent lives should not be sacrificed to make room for a returning older brother or sister. Preparation is the surest antidote to avoid resentment of an old face returning to the household and create a welcoming atmosphere where your adult child can be expected to return in kind.
- **Be a parent:** Your adult child may need more than a roof over their head. Some young people mature later than others, and their return to the nest could be based more on social anxiety or loneliness issues. Even as you welcome them back into the fold, you need to determine all the dynamics involved here and encourage them to get professional help if their moving back is rooted in more than purely financial reasons. Additionally, suppose the inability to manage their financial situation is their sole reason for living with you. In that case, they need to develop a plan to remedy that since living at home is not a viable long-term solution.

# PART SEVEN
# RELATIONSHIPS

*We are afraid to care too much, for fear that the other person does not care at all.*

—ELEANOR ROOSEVELT

*The great actress Katharine Hepburn once said, "Sometimes I wonder if men and women really suit each other. Perhaps they should live next door and just visit now and then."*

*Given the number of patients I've seen who are struggling in their marriages, I guess I can't argue with her. Relationships can be the greatest thing in someone's life or the primary cause of stress and angst—sometimes, they can be both at the same time.*

*I had a sixty-five-year-old female patient I was seeing because of anxiety she was feeling over the blended family she was trying to make work. Both she and her partner not only had adult children, but they also both had grandchildren. And the man had two high school–aged children from a second marriage my patient was now sharing the house with, and they didn't get along with her adult children, who both had young kids.*

*The woman was fixating on everything that went wrong and blamed herself for it all, most notably the conflicts she took entirely upon herself to resolve. When her stepchildren fought, she blamed herself. She blamed herself when there was a conflict with her own children and her new family. My work with her centered on the proposition that conflict was natural and okay, and she shouldn't feel she needed to fix everything.*

*"But it's my family," she said to me. "Shouldn't I take responsibility?"*

*We discussed her doing that by helping to resolve conflict instead of putting all the responsibility for fixing it on herself. During therapy, she also realized that her husband took the opposite approach by choosing to sit out these conflicts and that since he wasn't doing his part, she had taken on the onus of doing it for both of them.*

*She was doing too much, and he wasn't doing enough. My patient never confronted her husband on that out of concern it would damage their relationship. Still, the realization on its own helped her begin to deal with conflict differently so it came to stop dominating her life.*

# TROUBLED MARRIAGES

A husband and his wife came to see me a few years back to help them deal with their troubled marriage. I asked them why they wanted to stay together, and they both said, in so many words, for the children's sake.

"Okay," I said, "give me another reason why you want to remain married."

They looked at each other, hemmed and hawed, but ultimately couldn't give me one viable reason to stay together other than their kids.

"I think you should get divorced," I told them.

I do believe couples therapy can do great things when you have two partners who genuinely want to work things out. First off, I don't think the majority of people stay in troubled marriages because of the children. They stay together because neither of the spouses can recognize that their marriage is effectively over, so they foist everything onto their kids, and that's not a rational thing to do. It serves no one's betterment or happiness.

The first thing I might ask patients who come to me with marital problems is how they are different from their wedding day. How have they changed, grown, and evolved? "Well then," I might say to them, "has your partner done the same?" Almost inevitably, their answer is yes.

My point in doing this is that neither partner is the same person they were however many years ago when they got married. For marriages to work in the long term, the partners must grow vertically on parallel tracks, not tracks that diverge to the point where they barely even recognize each other. All people deserve to be happy, and I have seen far too many people over the years who stay in marriages that make them miserable. Often, they come to me because they want to try to work the problems out and fix things, and almost invariably, I'll agree with that and seek to help them in the effort. However, once my patients have tried everything for months or even years, they might ask me what else they can do. The mere fact they're posing that question tells me they already know the answer.

When they ask me what they can do to save their marriage in our first or another early session, here's some of the counsel I give them and what to be wary of.

## PRESCRIPTIONS FOR A TROUBLED MARRIAGE

- **Commitment:** They have to genuinely want, in their hearts and minds, for the marriage to work and be willing to do whatever it takes to make that happen. The problem is it literally does take two to tango, and both partners must share the same commitment. It will seldom work when a single partner takes the responsibility alone, because it isn't a single partner bringing the marriage down.

- **Responsibility:** Similarly, both partners need to acknowledge responsibility for the current state of their relationship to improve it. Marriage is a car with two steering wheels, not one, and too many couples end up driving into a ditch and blaming each other for the accident. By its very nature, marriage is a shared experience, and the responsibility for the partners' current plight must also be shared.
- **Communication:** Good, positive communication cures all, right? Unfortunately, this is not the case in troubled marriages because, again, both partners must be willing to change how they talk to each other. If only one expresses their feelings, it could push them further apart instead of closer together. You have to acknowledge that both of you have changed and what used to work from a communication standpoint may not work anymore. The prescription for that is to, first, acknowledge it and, second, accept that staying together means developing a different practice of communication between you and your partner.
- **Expectations:** We touched on this earlier, but, with few exceptions, partners shouldn't expect their marriages to be one long honeymoon. Instead, they should expect the change that comes with the passing of the years—their children growing up and moving on, facing financial and workplace challenges, and potentially meeting someone who seems to make them happier. They might still love each other but need to adjust their expectations about what that love means in the

present as opposed to the past. Believe it or not, some of the most enduring marriages I've seen in my patients are between two people who stay together because they believe the alternative will be worse. Their expectations have changed with the years.

- **Marital exercises:** I have suggested to patients who want to stay married that maybe they should take a trip together, just the two of them. Something like a cruise, somewhere tropical, adventurous, or exotic—so long as it's something they both enjoy. I might ask them what they enjoyed doing together the most when they were young. If they say camping, for example, I suggest they try that to rekindle the spark between them. Here's the thing, though: The spark might not ignite the same fire as before, but any fire can be a foundation to rebuild their relationship or construct a new one based on who they are in the moment. A January 2025 article in the Science Times section of *The New York Times* proposed a principle called "Commit to Joy," in which the article recommended, "Once a month or so, sit down with your partner and jot down three things each of you would like to do together.... Then swap lists. Take one item from your partner's list (and vice versa) and commit to helping make it happen."[78]
- **Go deeper:** Sometimes, the basis for marital strife can be as basic as one partner catching the other having an affair or that partner coming clean about it. Most times that strife has deep-seated roots. I often hear the term "loveless marriage" being thrown around, but I don't use it. Marriages can survive without love or a different definition of love, but they can't survive without

respect and acceptance. Psychotherapy can be a great way to identify and deal with the underlying issues because it prevents one or both partners from sticking their heads in the sand. You have to be able to look at yourself honestly and objectively if you're going to regard your partner the same way.

- **Patience:** Things didn't go off the rails overnight, and it will take a while to get back on them. There are no quick fixes or magical pills. Patience allows the partners to acknowledge and enjoy small victories together, like celebrating their child's wedding, graduation, bar/bat mitzvah, or confirmation. Milestones like these remind them that there was plenty of good before things went bad, and maybe that fact alone is enough to make them realize it's worth the time it takes to try to get things right and feel good like that again.

# DIVORCE

Some marriages can't be saved or can only be saved by one or both partners sacrificing their happiness. And for those marriages, divorce is not something to be shunned but embraced as a necessity.

I'm seeing more and more patients who divorce after their kids finish school and leave the home. Sometimes it's because the kids were the only thing holding the marriage together, something the partners may not have even realized until then that it was falling apart. In other instances, it's because empty nesters tend to reevaluate their priorities and mentally catalog where they are in life and where they want to be, independent of their children. Interestingly, some of the divorces that result from that are the most bitter and contested of any, even though custody and child support have left the picture. After all, there are usually more resources, money, and possessions to divvy up.

Believe it or not, though, according to a March 2024 article on CNN Health, marriage and divorce rates are declining.

"Being stuck in a home together during [COVID] lockdown forced a lot of couples to face problems in their relationship head-on," the article said, paraphrasing licensed marriage and family therapist Marissa Nelson. "That might have caused additional strife or helped them lay better groundwork for a stable future. Changes over the past two decades may also have helped. Therapy has become more normalized, marriage roles have become more flexible, and people are more used to talking openly about how they want their marriages to work."[79]

Like many topics this book covers, no two divorces are the same. Additionally, men and women face different dynamics. Let's take a frank and realistic look at all that.

## PRESCRIPTIONS FOR MANAGING DIVORCE

- **Take care of yourself:** I've harped on this repeatedly, but you need to be especially cognizant of it when managing the stress of going through a divorce. The process can be all-consuming. You may feel let down and betrayed, and your life may no longer be on the glide path it has followed for any number of years. As a result, you may also feel like crawling into a hole and burying yourself. Don't. This is the time you need to prioritize self-care even more than usual. Get to the gym, keep to your exercise routine, eat well, and strive in those moments to not let the process drag you down. The best prescription for staying as positive as you can is to focus as much as possible on activities you enjoy with the people you enjoy being with.
- **Compartmentalization:** Unfortunately, I've had patients who've brought the whole process into the workplace, becoming less productive and letting their looming divorce consume their lives. I work with them

on how best to compartmentalize what they're experiencing so they don't lose even more than a spouse. You don't want the remaining pillars of your life to suffer from the emotional turmoil you're experiencing. Your work can be a positive distraction from that upheaval, because it's something that's still going to be there after the divorce is completed, representing stability in unstable times. There's a show called *Severance* on Apple TV in which the home and work lives of the characters are scientifically cut off from each other. While that's not possible in the real world, dragging the baggage of your personal life into work can be even worse than the reverse.

- **Advice of counsel:** Few divorces are resolved amicably by cooperative partners. Unfortunately, the majority are contentious to varying degrees and require the involvement of attorneys on both sides to deal with disputes over the division of resources, alimony, and, depending on the age of the children, custody, which is often the most fraught issue of all. That means your choice of lawyer will be among the most important decisions you ever make. Ask friends for referrals and interview as many candidates as possible to find the lawyer with whom you feel most comfortable for your situation.
- **The kids:** If the kids are still school-age, even in college, your challenge here will obviously be greater. Unfortunately, the more contentious the divorce, the harder it becomes to keep the children out of it. I've heard from patients all the time how their soon-to-be former spouse is turning the kids against them. Their instinct is to respond in kind, but I advise them as much as

possible to avoid that, because tit-for-tat serves no one's best interests. That's why it's vital to keep the lines of communication open. If a separation has removed you from the household, maintaining quality time with your kids is the best way to ensure that it continues after the divorce is finalized. It will also allow you and them to get used to the new lifestyle you will all be experiencing. I've found that being strong for your kids can be an excellent prescription for finding the strength in yourself you'll need to get through this.

- **Support system:** In addition to psychotherapy, which may be warranted to help you come to grips with your feelings, you need others to help get you through the process emotionally. Your "normal" has been ripped away, and you need to compensate for that by finding a new normal that doesn't entail you wallowing in your pain. Support groups, both in-person and online, exist too, and it is worth trying to see if sharing your experiences and listening to others relate theirs might be right for you. Spend as much time as you can with family and friends, and remember that much of what you've taken for granted, like celebrating holidays and birthdays together, won't be there anymore. You need to construct a new normal for yourself, which means not clinging to the expectations of the old one and building a support system that will help you adapt to the new life you'll be waking up to every morning.
- **Preparation:** *I just can't believe they did… I never expected them to… Can you believe that…* These are all common refrains patients express before they relate some form of betrayal, duplicity, or vindictive behavior

on the part of their spouses. While I do commiserate with them, I'm also prone to saying something to the effect that this shouldn't surprise them, and such actions by their spouse shouldn't shock them either. I advise patients going through divorce to expect to be unpleasantly surprised. That, however, doesn't always do much good when they're confronted with outright lies and absurd demands regarding money and custody. Just because things start in a fairly amicable way doesn't mean they're going to stay that way, and you need to prepare yourself for that.

- **Resources:** "The average cost of a divorce in the United States ranges between $15,000 and $20,000, but it can vary dramatically depending on the level of enmity between the couple, whether the couple had children and even the state they reside in."[80] I've had patients who spend three, four, even five times that to ultimately arrive at the same resolution they could have at the outset with a handshake. The primary cause for this is the animus that has developed between the couple or one partner toward the other. It almost feels like they don't just want to move on; they want to ruin their soon-to-be former partner's life in the process. Divorce is inevitably contentious, but it doesn't have to be spiteful and vindictive, and the best way to keep the process on track is by keeping an eye on the bottom line of the resources you're expending often for naught.

# FINDING A NEW PARTNER (IF YOU WANT ONE)

These days, people coming out of relationships for whatever reason have a multitude of options for starting over again. This process means something different to everyone based on their needs, expectations, and age.

Men and women seeking a fresh start, or a restart, in life have various options. For some, it could mean reconnecting with someone from their past. For others, it could be finding a partner but not a spouse. For still more, it's finding a companion who, like you, wishes to live separately and maintain their individual lives while also being a couple—call that having your cake and eating it too. It's one I'm seeing more and more in my patients, particularly in those around Social Security age. For these and others, falling head over heels in love again is neither a desire nor a possibility. Yet it opens up so many experiences when you have someone to share them with; no matter how you define the relationship, it will enrich the latter years of your life.

Younger people may find this road more challenging to travel than older ones. For older individuals, the notion of child-rearing has mostly been left in the past. Both partners will likely have their own children and even grandchildren. So their relationship is not so much about starting over as picking up in the middle and enjoying life in the company of someone who shares the same goals as they do in that regard.

Younger folks, on the other hand, may be looking to start another family, which can potentially lead to complications in its own right. If one or both of the partners have older children from an earlier relationship, those kids may not accept significantly younger siblings into their lives. Raising young children means the respective partners will have less time and resources to spend on the children from their last relationship. I've also had patients tell me of the financial struggles they face when burning resources to raise their new family while still paying child support to the old one.

Let's look at the mental checklist you should perform before pursuing a new partner.

## PRESCRIPTIONS FOR FINDING A NEW PARTNER

- **Know your priorities:** Carefully consider what you're looking for to maximize the opportunity to find someone whose priorities match yours. In that regard, make sure you're honest with yourself, and don't think you should change your intentions just because you find someone you like. Or, better yet, ask yourself if this person is worth reconsidering the priorities you set when embarking on this path.

- **Be honest with yourself:** I have patients who can't be happy unless they're in a relationship and patients who are much happier on their own. As a psychotherapist, I try to get them to understand their feelings and realize a situation that's great for someone else isn't necessarily a good fit for them. Some patients I've seen want to be in a relationship because they hate being alone, and I try to help them work on getting in better touch with themselves first before committing to someone else again.
- **Learn to trust your instincts:** When coming out of a relationship, you must rely on instincts you haven't used in years. That, though, doesn't change the fact there's nothing better than your gut to tell you if you've met the right person. Patients ask me how they can be sure. After telling them there are no hard-and-fast rules, I mention some behaviors that will help inform them. Do they have to choose their words carefully, or is the conversation natural, especially over a lengthy dinner? Can they name three things they have in common with their potential new partner? What attracted them to the person in the first place? When they say looks, I worry. I smile when they say smile, personality, or meeting over a shared interest.
- **Cast your net:** There are many ways people meet their potential new partners, but in my experience, an introduction from a mutual friend or casual acquaintance yields the highest percentage of success. People like that already know both of you. I have a patient, for example, who was introduced to the second love of his life by their mutual divorce lawyer. But the lawyer never

would have made the introduction in the first place if they hadn't known my patient was looking to meet someone. The more people who know that in your life, the more likely you will find who you're looking for. In this case, your support system becomes your wingman or woman.

- **Take your time:** Rushing into a relationship just for the sake of it is a recipe for failure. If you're miserable alone and willing to settle, you need to take a step back and make sure you've shed the baggage left over from your last relationship. That will also give you time to rebuild your confidence and self-esteem. Sometimes, I might add, you find exactly who you're looking for when you're not trying. Being patient increases the odds of finding that person naturally and organically.
- **Social media:** Social media and dating apps, appropriately used, can be a great tool for finding someone, the best of all for many individuals. And that process comes with the added benefit of taking a systematic approach to the whole process. However, the convenience of social media brings inherent dangers, which you must be aware of before you start scrolling through names and faces. That's why I've dedicated the entire next chapter to social media.

# SOCIAL MEDIA

Many who turn to social media sites and dating apps don't have the skill or savvy to discern what may be lurking behind a person's profile. As I said earlier, I am amazed at how many people use the internet to find relationships and how many of these relationships actually work. Appropriately used, these apps can be a fantastic tool in which relationships can start based on a simple comment to a post or picture, perhaps about something you have in common with the person.

Maybe both of you have three kids. Or root for the same sports team. Or come from the same area. Or enjoy the same movies, TV shows, or books. The list is endless and can be a great conversation starter, if nothing else. This approach isn't for everybody, but there's no harm in trying as long as you educate yourself on the broad scope of what the internet offers in this respect. It can't hurt to message someone who feels right to you, just to see if there might be something there.

While social media sites can be great resources and boast any number of success stories, they come with a dark side populated by scammers, frauds, and con artists who can completely upend or even ruin your life. For some reason, people don't always practice the same caution from the distance of cyberspace they do from up close and personal.

As *The New York Times* reported in August 2024, a retired corporate executive lost $100,000 in one such targeted scam. Splashing his vulnerability across social media was like ringing the dinner bell for hungry scam farms based in third-world countries across the globe in a process known as "catfishing," which entails creating a false identity online for the purposes of deception. In this case, the target was fodder for a nonexistent banker named Alice, who won his trust and attention as a prelude to coaxing him into investing his money in Bitcoin.

"But when he went to withdraw his fictitious winnings from what he later realized was a phony trading app," wrote Tara Siegel Bernard in that *New York Times* article, "the platform told him that his account was frozen because of potential money laundering—and that he would have to pay to release it. When he told the trading app that he would contact the F.B.I., [the woman] vanished."[81]

Recovering your money from any of these scam farms is virtually impossible.

"Dennis Jones, an avid runner and photographer, was adored by his children and grandchildren," CNN reported in another tragic example. "Described as 'a bit of an activist' by his family, the 82-year-old spent much of his retirement working with refugees and debating politics online. But in the last few months of his life, he withdrew from his family and, having been divorced for years, befriended a woman named Jessie on Facebook. The two had been talking online for months and built a close relationship. Eventually, Jessie convinced Dennis to invest in crypto. Dennis complied. He spent everything he had without ever meeting Jessie in person, and when he had nothing left, she demanded more. Until one day, the money disappeared, leaving him in ruin."[82]

Not long after, Dennis took his own life.

In another catfishing romance scam, a case featured on *Dr. Phil* involved a woman named Sarah who was scammed out of $1.4 million by a man she had never met. Believing she was in a genuine online romance, Sarah sent large sums of money to someone who convinced her he was her boyfriend. Even after Dr. Phil and investigators revealed the truth, and she was confronted with the real person whose identity had been stolen, Sarah struggled to accept it. Despite the overwhelming evidence, she held on to the hope that her relationship was real.[83]

So how can you avoid becoming a victim of social media like Sarah?

## PRESCRIPTIONS FOR AVOIDING SOCIAL MEDIA SCAMS

- **Verify their identity:** Before you embark on a relationship, research and verify the person's identity through other social media sites, Google searches, or even paying a nominal amount for a criminal background check. If you don't find anything, the person likely doesn't exist.
- **Be suspicious:** If the relationship progresses too quickly, you should see a flashing yellow light warning you to slow down. Tell your new friend it's time to meet up in person. If they resist or make excuses, the light should change to red.

- **Red flags:** If your new potential partner asks you for money for any reason, investment or otherwise, find someone else. That's just not normal social behavior. Beware also of them feeding you a sob story about having a sick kid or being sick themselves, which might otherwise lead you to offer them money to help. The number of people who continue to fall prey to such scams astounds me, indicative of someone so desperate to meet someone that their gullibility trumps everything else.
- **Guard personal information:** Although I have never had a patient admit to me that they were scammed this way, I remain amazed at how often smart people share their personal or financial information with virtual strangers they only know from chatting or messaging online.
- **Educate yourself:** It will only take a small bit of research to educate yourself on the latest social media romance scams that are out there. Remember, you're not the first potential victim. Forewarned, as the saying goes, is forearmed.
- **Know your enemy:** These romance scammers are experts at preying on vulnerabilities. Be especially leery when a potential match reaches out to you first. If everything about that person is too perfect, if they check every box, your suspicions should be raised.

# FOR MEN ONLY

There are many reasons why older men are attracted to younger women, most prominently the opportunity to defy Father Time and feel young again. As Marriage.com posted in March 2024, "[The younger woman's] energy and lust for life will, in all likelihood, transfer over to you, the older man. This has a positive effect on your health and well-being. Your younger wife will not be content to sit at home binge-watching the latest series on Netflix. She will get you out of your armchair and back into the world. Before, your weekends weren't very exciting. Now, she wants you to rock out at Coachella with her, and why not book a trek in the Himalayas? Her enthusiasm to explore and discover the world is contagious, making you see and experience things with fresh eyes."[84]

That rosy picture of a growing trend, especially among men of means and opportunity, taints the primary reason why age-gap relationships appeal to younger women: men can father children into their sixties, seventies, and even their eighties.

But does that make it a good idea?

While every case is different, there are some universal truths about age-gap relationships yielding children. Becoming a father again when many of your peers, and potentially even yourself, already have grandchildren may seem appealing because it can feel like a sip from the Fountain of Youth. Unfortunately, that sip often comes with a sour aftertaste. If your child is born when you're sixty, you'll go to soccer games and parent-teacher conferences well into your seventies. And if your child is born when you're seventy, or eighty…

Math doesn't lie. Many men who choose or agree to have children later in life have often forgotten how hard and time-consuming it was the first time around, assuming there was one. You also may find that the younger woman you've fallen in love with will not be the same woman you committed yourself to once she's left to devote herself to her newborn. Her priorities and passion will be rerouted to the point where the relationship might drastically change, leading to a potential breach if your expectations aren't redefined with your child's birth. Your younger partner may not want to go out much for a considerable stretch, and any travel plans you have entertained will likely have to be placed on hold.

You may have adult children already, so you need to ask yourself how they will respond to having a half brother or sister decades their junior. Is it worth potentially breaching that relationship or driving a wedge between you?

The question may be moot because, even if you've exercised caution upon entering this arena, you may reluctantly agree to become a father again so you don't lose the younger woman you've fallen head over heels for and has transformed your life for the better. In other cases, I have observed the man has been a willing partner because he feels this will be his last opportunity at fatherhood. In many of these cases, though, he doesn't really know what he's in for.

If you find yourself going down the road of an age-gap relationship, what are the most important things to keep in mind?

## PRESCRIPTIONS FOR MEN INVOLVED WITH YOUNGER WOMEN

- **Consider a prenuptial agreement:** In my experience, schisms with younger children from previous marriages are more likely to arise over money than bearing children. Every man has the right to be happy. But suppose his younger partner's feelings for him are genuine. In that case, she will not object to a reasonable agreement that leaves her, and any children, well cared for without necessarily reaping most or all of her older partner's estate upon his passing.
- **Talk to your other children:** There is no worse approach than springing the news of your commitment to an age-gap relationship on your adult children. Instead, you should appropriately bring them into the fold and, potentially, at least try to make your new partner a part of their extended family. Keeping the relationship and your intentions secret leads to resentment and potential recriminations about the woman's motivations. If her motivations truly mirror yours, you should not be reluctant to keep your adult children fully in the loop about something that will affect their lives.
- **Don't prejudge:** On the other hand, I've also had patients who express discomfort to me about what the younger woman who has come into their lives may be after. While these concerns are wholly justified, they do

not inherently mean that the young woman's attraction to you is not every bit as real as your attraction to her. Younger women, especially those who may have experienced difficult relationships in the past, might very well be looking for stability and financial security in their lives. The notion of a "daddy figure" who offers maturity, guidance, and a sense of authority can appeal to women considerably younger than the man they've become attracted to.

- **Acknowledge the realities:** Understand that you're likely not going to be around for the milestones of life younger parents get to celebrate. Depending on your age and health, be honest with yourself about whether you'll be alive when the child graduates from high school, never mind college. In all probability, you won't be there for their wedding or the birth of their children. And know that you will spend the rest of your life in the company of parents who may be younger than your own adult children and, in some cases, even closer to your grandchildren's ages.
- **What's in it for you:** Some men don't want to be alone, no matter their age. They've never been alone, and they never want to be alone. Take ninety-three-year-old Rupert Murdoch, for example. As the *Sydney Morning Herald* reported in March 2023, "He married Anna Torv a year after he divorced his first wife, and Wendi Deng three weeks after he divorced Torv. He had a two-year break between Deng and Jerry Hall, but met his new fiancée Ann-Lesley Smith just one month after divorcing Hall." [85] There's also comfort for some older men in having a built-in caretaker as the

inevitable declines associated with age set in. That may not be the ideal foundation for building a relationship, but it's reality.

- **Is it fair to the child:** Along with the health risks when older men conceive children, there's also the very real possibility of the child growing up no longer with the active presence of a father, or without a father at all, very early in their lives. That is a moral dilemma the partners in any age-gap relationship must face. The decision is theirs alone, but it should be made with a realistic view of the consequences that their decision might very well yield.

# FOR WOMEN ONLY

A female patient, and mother herself, once told me of passing a table in a restaurant where a younger man was dining with an older woman.

"How wonderful to see a mother and her son enjoying quality time together," she said, smiling warmly.

"Ma'am," said the young man, "this is my girlfriend."

My patient walked away with her foot in her mouth, completely embarrassed.

The dynamics of relationships between older women and younger men, so-called cougar relationships, are entirely different from the reverse. But they're the same in one significant way: Everyone deserves the opportunity to be happy, so long as they're not hurting anyone else. A relationship with an older woman may be unthinkable for most younger men, but that doesn't make it wrong for a young man who finds fulfillment and enrichment in one.

Of course, the biggest distinction between the older man–younger woman dynamic is that the reverse never involves having a child since the woman is past childbearing age and the younger man may not be interested in being a father. Not a lot of attention is paid to this trend, which is more common than you think. Typically, discussion is spurred by the likes of Ashton Kutcher and his relationship with Demi Moore, who was fifteen years his senior. Or the media fetish over the fact that French President Emmanuel Macron's spouse Brigitte is twenty-four years older than him.

Writing in *Psychology Today* in March 2023 about a study he conducted, Dr. Justin Lehmiller said, "What I found was that women who were more than 10 years older than their male partners were actually the most satisfied with and committed to their relationships compared with both women who were younger than their partners, as well as women whose partners were close in age. In other words, in spite of the stigma associated with older women dating younger men, the women in these relationships were thriving on average."[86]

Unfortunately, the same social stigma doesn't seem to apply to relationships between older men and younger women, and there's no associated term like "cougar" to suggest similarly negative connotations. Far too many people find power in looking disparagingly on and judging others. Putting someone else down somehow seems to lift them up. However, among the recurring themes of this book is to each their own. The human psyche doesn't come with an owner's manual. Different fuels power the needs and desires of different people, all helping us get to whatever we define as fulfillment.

If you are a woman in this kind of relationship, it's wise to educate yourself on what to expect and how to maximize the chances for the relationship to flourish.

## PRESCRIPTIONS FOR WOMEN ONLY

- **Companionship:** There is nothing wrong with an older woman forming a relationship or partnership with a younger man. After all, the partners in the relationship are seeking the same thing traditional partners do: attaining a level of happiness that is enhanced and defined by their being together. However, I have found in my patients that the most important factor in successful age-gap relationships is how much they simply enjoy each other's company. They were friends and companions before they became partners, friends before they may have become lovers.
- **Communication:** Even more so than same general age relationships, age-gap partnerships require the partners to be open and honest with each other. The partners may not share as much in common in terms of interests, goals, and concerns, but the strength of their bond can overcome all that, so long as neither partner feels deceived, let down, or misled at any point. It's wise to remember that participants in an age-gap relationship may very well be more sensitive to the issues and challenges all relationships face because of the pressure over their deviation from societal norms.
- **Expectations:** Defining the parameters of the relationship between an older woman and a younger man is vital. What if he has younger friends he still wants to spend time with, and how does that mesh socially? After all, it isn't realistic to expect the couple to fit in with the couples closer to his age. So, too, it's unrealistic

to expect the reverse to be true, and the couple must face the fact that social norms will render continuing relationships with people in each partner's respective age group a difficult hill to climb.

- **Overcoming challenges:** The younger man's parents will almost surely be around the same age, or even younger, than his partner. And the older woman's children may very well be about the same age or younger than her partner. So their relationship is likely to strain long-term relationships with, and even stoke resentment and alienation from, family members. Hopefully, this can and will resolve over time with patience, but be aware that isn't always the case.
- **Mutual respect:** In successful age-gap relationships, nothing is more important than the mutual respect each partner maintains for the interests, preferences, choices, opinions, and desires of the other. Such respect acts as a shield to help insulate the partners from naysayers and antagonists, and if your bond is strong enough, you'll be able to withstand any outside threats to your relationship.
- **Realities:** Not everyone will accept your relationship, and the reaction of many friends or family members may be vitriolic. If you feel strongly enough for each other, you will be able to overcome this, but it may require sacrifice. The younger man must also face the reality that he will still be relatively young or middle-aged when the older woman is aging into a situation where her care needs are changing and evolving. "'Til death do us part" bears an entirely different meaning in any age-gap relationship, and the younger partner

must be able to come to terms with eventually becoming the older partner's caregiver, left to deal with adult children potentially he may not be on the best of terms with among the other responsibilities and hardships he accepted when he entered into the relationship.

# EPILOGUE

*Once you replace negative thoughts with positive ones, you'll start having positive results.*

—WILLIE NELSON

I began this book by telling you a little about myself and that I want you to build the happiest, most rewarding, and fullest life possible. In that sense, seven sections and forty-three topics later, *The Myth of Aging* is like a toolbox to help you achieve that. You won't need to use all the tools inside, but hopefully you found the right ones that apply most directly to the task at hand.

I started this book by presenting ten **Do I** questions and advising that if you answered yes to two or more of them, this book would help you or someone close to you. Let's try that exercise again:

- Do I wake up in the morning feeling poorly physically or emotionally?
- Do I eat poorly?
- Do I sleep poorly?

- Do I wish my relationships were more fulfilling?
- Do I wish I was happier?
- Do I want to be a better person?
- Do I want to change places with someone else?
- Do I have little to look forward to?
- Do I wish I could do things over again?
- Do I have a lot of regrets?

I hope your answers are all no's this time or, at the very least, you've made progress. Because mental and emotional health improvements often move in inches instead of feet. I tell my patients their goal should be to feel a little better at a time about themselves and their daily lives, to measure their progress in feet instead of yards. To help you do that, here are the prescriptions that appeared most often in these pages in general, all-encompassing terms:

- **Acceptance:** Before we can expect the world to accept us as we are, we have to accept ourselves and be willing to change if we don't like what we figuratively see in the mirror. Try to see yourself as others see you, and never stop seeking strategies for self-improvement.
- **Self-Care:** If you don't take care of yourself, nothing else matters. To maximize your happiness and capacity to be fulfilled by life, you need to exercise, eat right, and get enough rest. These need to be priorities, not afterthoughts as they are for far too many people.
- **Patience:** Everyone wants immediate gratification, but life's most important and lasting things don't come that way. There is no expiration date for your goals, and if the road you're on hasn't taken you where you want to go, consider mentally rerouting yourself.

- **Communication:** I wholeheartedly believe that misunderstanding or miscommunication is the root cause of most squabbles, conflicts, and breakdowns in relationships. Make sure to express your feelings clearly and succinctly. When applicable, this applies to your partner, kids, superiors, associates, peers, friends, clients, and co-workers. Make your feelings and where you stand clear so no one can misinterpret what you say or write.
- **Support:** Everyone needs a shoulder to squeeze or cry on, just as everyone needs to know they have reliable friends and relatives who will be there for them no matter what, people whose company you genuinely enjoy and who will have your back when you need them the most. So, too, nothing makes a person feel better than the ability to be there for someone else they care about. It cuts both ways.
- **Resilience:** No one gets through life unscathed. Life is messy, and everyone gets knocked down from time to time. You can't be as happy or successful as you want without getting up fast and moving on. That's not always easy, but it's a big part of happiness and fulfillment.
- **Attitude:** Attitude matters. If you don't believe you can accomplish something, you start with a distinct disadvantage. Just because you do believe doesn't assure success, but it does assure much higher odds of achieving what you want in both your personal and professional lives. And the better your attitude, the better you'll be able to deal with adversity. The obstacles life throws in your path will feel more like rocks than boulders.

- **Psychotherapy:** This book is not intended to be a replacement for psychotherapy for those who feel they'd be better served by having a professional to help them work out the issues that brought them to its pages. Remember to seek out a therapist with whom you can quickly establish rapport and trust and whose feedback steers you in the direction that encourages you to accomplish your goals.

I recommend that you make a copy, or screenshot, of the list above and place it where you have to look at it every day as a reminder of what you need to do to continue feeling better about yourself and knowing how to find happiness. Hopefully, you'll hear my voice when you think about what you want out of life and how to use these tools to best achieve it.

The fee for this session was no more than the price of this book, the content of which you can revisit time and time again. Always remember, though, that life is neither a sprint nor a marathon. It's a roller coaster, with a mix of dips and darts, highs and lows, hits and misses, and wins that can make the losses pale by comparison.

My final prescription for you is to strap yourself in and enjoy the ride.

# ENDNOTES

## PART ONE: PHYSICAL AND MENTAL FITNESS

1 "Our Epidemic of Loneliness and Isolation: The U.S. Surgeon General's Advisory on the Healing Effects of Social Connection and Community," report issued in 2023 by the Department of Health and Human Services (https://www.hhs.gov/sites/default/files/surgeon-general-social-connection-advisory.pdf).

2 "Older Men's Connections Often Wither When They're on Their Own," Judith Graham, KFF News; October 10, 2024 (https://kffhealthnews.org/news/article/older-men-connections-isolation-loneliness-navigating-aging/).

3 "Learn How to Avoid Romance Scams," Dierdre van Dyk, AARP; updated February 4, 2025 (https://www.aarp.org/money/scams-fraud/romance/).

4 "Physical Activity Among Adults Aged 18 and Over: United States, 2020," report issued by the CDC's National Center for Health Statistics, August 2022 (https://www.cdc.gov/nchs/products/databriefs/db443.htm).

5 "Physical Activity Guidelines for Americans, 2nd edition," report issued by the Department of Health and Human Services in 2018 (https://odphp.health.gov/sites/default/files/2019-09/Physical_Activity_Guidelines_2nd_edition.pdf).

6 "Child Activity: An Overview," report issued by the Centers for Disease Control in January 2024 (https://www.cdc.gov/physical-activity-basics/guidelines/children.html).

7 "Women Get Less Exercise Than Men. It's a Problem," Danielle Freeman, *New York Times*; November 19, 2024.

8 "Special Report: Using Nutrition as a Therapeutic Modality," Marta Mudd, PhD, *Psychiatric News*; January 18, 2025 (https://psychiatryonline.org/doi/10.1176/appi.pn.2025.01.1.18).

9 "Obesity and Severe Obesity Prevalence in Adults: United States, August 2021–August 2023," report issued by the CDC's National Center for Health Statistics, August 2022 (https://www.cdc.gov/nchs/products/databriefs/db508.htm).

10 "The Psychological Burden of Obesity," report issued by the National Institute of Health's National Library of Medicine, July 2018 (https://pmc.ncbi.nlm.nih.gov/articles/PMC6052856/).

11 "Special Report: Using Nutrition as a Therapeutic Modality," Marta Mudd, PhD, *Psychiatric News*; January 18, 2025 (https://psychiatryonline.org/doi/10.1176/appi.pn.2025.01.1.18).

12 "Special Report: Using Nutrition as a Therapeutic Modality," Marta Mudd, PhD, *Psychiatric News*; January 18, 2025 (https://psychiatryonline.org/doi/10.1176/appi.pn.2025.01.1.18).

13 "35 Simple Health Tips Experts Swear By," Amanda Schupak, *New York Times*; January 12, 2025 (https://www.nytimes.com/interactive/2025/01/12/well/health-tips-experts.html).

14 "What Is Mindfulness? A Simple Practice for Greater Well-being," Crystal Hoshaw, Healthline; March 29, 2022 (https://www.healthline.com/health/mind-body/what-is-mindfulness).

15 "Mindfulness," American Psychological Association, adapted from APA Dictionary of Psychology, April 2018 (https://www.apa.org/topics/mindfulness).

16 "Study: Mindfulness Meditation Works as Well as Common Antidepressant to Reduce Anxiety," Kaitlin Sullivan, *Health*; November 16, 2022 (https://www.health.com/mindfulness-meditation-antidepressant-reduce-anxiety-6828775).

17 "Study: Mindfulness Meditation Works as Well as Common Antidepressant to Reduce Anxiety," Kaitlin Sullivan, *Health*; November 16, 2022 (https://www.health.com/mindfulness-meditation-antidepressant-reduce-anxiety-6828775).

18 "What Is Mindfulness? A Simple Practice for Greater Well-being," Crystal Hoshaw, Healthline; March 29, 2022 (https://www.healthline.com/health/mind-body/what-is-mindfulness).

## PART TWO: RESILIENCE

19 "Speaking of Psychology: The Stress of Money, with Linda Gallo, PhD," American Psychological Association, interview transcript (https://www.apa.org/news/podcasts/speaking-of-psychology/financial-stress).

20 "Coping with Financial Stress," Lawrence Robinson and Melinda Smith, MA, HelpGuide.org, undated (https://www.helpguide.org/mental-health/stress/coping-with-financial-stress).

21 "The Emotional Shock of Retirement," Stephanie Watson, WebMD; July 28, 2023 (https://www.webmd.com/healthy-aging/features/emotional-shock-retirement).

22 "The Relationship Between Spirituality and Resilience and Well-being," National Institute of Health, National Library of Medicine; February 11, 2023 (https://pmc.ncbi.nlm.nih.gov/articles/PMC9918825/).

23 "Building Resilience and Character Through Career Challenges: A Path to Professional Excellence," Pratik Kate, Medium; July 30, 2024 (https://katepratik.medium.com/building-resilience-and-character-through-career-challenges-a-path-to-professional-excellence-257c2787c38b).

## PART THREE: FINDING AND KEEPING HAPPINESS

24 "Less Than Half of Americans 'Very Satisfied' With Own Lives," Megan Brenan, Gallup; February 8, 2024 (https://news.gallup.com/poll/610133/less-half-americans-satisfied-own-lives.aspx).

25 "35 Simple Health Tips Experts Swear By," Amanda Schupak, *New York Times*; January 12, 2025 (https://www.nytimes.com/interactive/2025/01/12/well/health-tips-experts.html).

26 "35 Simple Health Tips Experts Swear By," Amanda Schupak, *New York Times*; January 12, 2025 (https://www.nytimes.com/interactive/2025/01/12/well/health-tips-experts.html).

27 "The Power of Pets: Health Benefits of Human-Animal Interactions," News in Health, National Institute of Health; February 2018 (https://newsinhealth.nih.gov/2018/02/power-pets).

28 "35 Simple Health Tips Experts Swear By," Amanda Schupak, *New York Times*; January 12, 2025 (https://www.nytimes.com/interactive/2025/01/12/well/health-tips-experts.html).

29 "Less than Half of Americans 'Very Satisfied' With Own Lives," Megan Brenan, Gallup; February 8, 2024 (https://news.gallup.com/poll/610133/less-half-americans-satisfied-own-lives.aspx).

## PART FOUR: COPING WITH TRAUMA

30 "Grief can hurt – in more ways than one: Stress and depression may lead to new health issues or intensify the symptoms of existing conditions," Harvard Health Publishing, Harvard Medical School; February 1, 2019 (https://www.health.harvard.edu/mind-and-mood/grief-can-hurt-in-more-ways-than-one).

31 "35 Simple Health Tips Experts Swear By," Amanda Schupak, *New York Times*; January 12, 2025 (https://www.nytimes.com/interactive/2025/01/12/well/health-tips-experts.html).

32 "Stay Active: Physical Decline Starts Earlier Than Thought," Cindy Sagon, AARP; August 25, 2016 (https://www.aarp.org/health/healthy-living/info-2016/fitness-aging-physical-decline-cs.html).

33 "Percentage of adults in the United States with select fears about aging as of 2024," Statista Research Department, Statista; February 15, 2024 (https://www.statista.com/statistics/1450999/share-of-adults-with-age-related-fears/).

34 "New Survey Reveals 87% of Americans have a Fear of Getting Old (FOGO) – Results Show Top Fear is Decline in Physical Ability," Pfizer Press Release; July 16, 2014 (https://www.pfizer.com/news/press-release/press-release-detail/fogo_new_survey_reveals_87_of_americans_have_a_fear_of_getting_old_fogo_results_show_top_fear_is_decline_in_physical_ability1).

35 "The Intensity and Effects of Strength Training in the Elderly," report issued by the National Library of Medicine, National Institute of Health; May 27, 2011 (https://pmc.ncbi.nlm.nih.gov/articles/PMC3117172/).

36 "The study of mindfulness as an intervening factor for enhanced psychological well-being in building the level of resilience," Vincent Kim Seng Oh, et al., National Institute of Health, National Library of Medicine; December 21, 2022 (https://pmc.ncbi.nlm.nih.gov/articles/PMC9811678/).

37 "Alcohol and aging – An area of increasing concern," Aaron M. White, et al., *Science Direct*; March 2023 (https://www.sciencedirect.com/science/article/abs/pii/S0741832922000660).

38 "The Cognitive Consequences of Alcohol Use," Ronald Devere, *Practical Neurology*; October 2016 (https://practicalneurology.com/articles/2016-oct/the-cognitive-consequences-of-alcohol-use#:~:text=Men%20who%20consumed%2036%20grams/day%20of%20alcohol,in%20global%20cognitive%20score%20and%20executive%20function).

39 "Antidepressant Use and Cognitive Decline: The Health and Retirement Study," National Library of Medicine, National Institute of Health; October 24, 2015 (https://pmc.ncbi.nlm.nih.gov/articles/PMC4618694/).

40 "In-Law Suites: A Growing Trend in Home Building," Neighborhoods.com; February 7, 2019 (https://www.neighborhoods.com/blog/in-law-suites-a-growing-trend-in-home-building).

41 "Adjustment Disorders," *The Mayo Clinic Press*; July 6, 2023 (https://www.mayoclinic.org/diseases-conditions/adjustment-disorders/symptoms-causes/syc-20355224).

42 "Prolonged Grief Disorder," reviewed by Paul Appelbaum, MD, and Lamyaa Yousiff, MD, PhD, MS, American Psychiatric Association; May 2022 (https://www.psychiatry.org/patients-families/prolonged-grief-disorder).

43 "What is Posttraumatic Stress Disorder (PTSD)," reviewed by Monica Taylor-Desir, MD, MPH, DFAPA, American Psychiatric Association; November 2022 (https://www.psychiatry.org/patients-families/ptsd/what-is-ptsd).

44 "Post traumatic stress disorder (PTSD)," Mind; January 2021 (https://www.mind.org.uk/information-support/types-of-mental-health-problems/post-traumatic-stress-disorder-ptsd-and-complex-ptsd/symptoms/).

45 "Cognitive Processing Therapy (CPT) for PTSD," U.S. Department of Veterans Affairs (https://www.ptsd.va.gov/understand_tx/cognitive_processing.asp).

46 "Prolonged Exposure (PE)," Clinical Practice Guideline for the Treatment of Posttraumatic Stress Disorder"; Updated June 2020 (https://www.apa.org/ptsd-guideline/treatments/prolonged-exposure).

47 "EMDR Therapy," *Cleveland Clinic*; March 29, 2022 (https://my.clevelandclinic.org/health/treatments/22641-emdr-therapy).

48 "In brief: Cognitive behavioral therapy (CBT)," report issued by the National Library of Medicine, National Institute of Health; June 2, 2022 (https://www.ncbi.nlm.nih.gov/books/NBK279297/).


## PART FIVE: YOUR INTIMATE SELF


49 "Sexual Activity and Physical Tenderness in Older Adults: Cross-Sectional Prevalence and Associated Characteristics," Roseanne Freak-Poli, et al., *Journal of Sexual Medicine*; July 2017 (https://www.researchgate.net/publication/318066593_Sexual_Activity_and_Physical_Tenderness_in_Older_Adults_Cross-Sectional_Prevalence_and_Associated_Characteristics).

50 "Teen Sexual Behavior," Quick Facts 2024: Sex Education in America, Ascend; August 12, 2024 (https://weascend.org/resource/quick-facts-2024-sex-education-in-america/).

51 "Study: Many Adults Ages 65 to 80 Continue to Be Sexually Active," Alexa Larieri. *U.S. News and World Report*; May 3, 2018 (https://www.usnews.com/news/health-care-news/articles/2018-05-03/study-many-adults-ages-65-to-80-continue-to-be-sexually-active).

52 "The Demographics of Remarriage," Gretchen Livingston, Pew Research Center; November 14, 2024 (https://www.pewresearch.org/social-trends/2014/11/14/chapter-2-the-demographics-of-remarriage/).

53 "35 Simple Health Tips Experts Swear By," Amanda Schupak, *New York Times*; January 12, 2025 (https://www.nytimes.com/interactive/2025/01/12/well/health-tips-experts.html).

54 "Live Sensibly, and Your Heart Will Thank You," Nina Agrawal, *New York Times*; January 14, 2025 (https://www.nytimes.com/2025/01/10/well/heart-disease-prevention.html?searchResultPosition=2).

55 "Live Sensibly, and Your Heart Will Thank You," Nina Agrawal, *New York Times*; January 14, 2025 (https://www.nytimes.com/2025/01/10/well/heart-disease-prevention.html?searchResultPosition=2).

56 "35 Simple Health Tips Experts Swear By," Amanda Schupak, *New York Times*; January 12, 2025 (https://www.nytimes.com/interactive/2025/01/12/well/health-tips-experts.html).

57 "LGBTQ+ Identification in U.S. Now at 7.6%," Jeffrey M. Jones, Gallup; March 13, 2024 (https://news.gallup.com/poll/611864/lgbtq-identification.aspx).

58 "Nearly 30% of Gen Z adults identify as LGBTQ, national survey finds," Matt Lavietes, NBC; January 24, 2024 (https://www.nbcnews.com/nbc-out/out-news/nearly-30-gen-z-adults-identify-lgbtq-national-survey-finds-rcna135510).

59 "Nearly 30% of Gen Z adults identify as LGBTQ, national survey finds," Matt Lavietes, NBC; January 24, 2024 (https://www.nbcnews.com/nbc-out/out-news/nearly-30-gen-z-adults-identify-lgbtq-national-survey-finds-rcna135510).

60 "Huntington Beach moves to Adopt Transgender & Sexuality Notification Law," Hosam Elattar, *Voice of OC*; September 4, 2024 (https://voiceofoc.org/2024/09/huntington-beach-moves-to-adopt-transgender-sexuality-notification-law/).

61 "LGBTQ People's Experiences of Workplace Discrimination and Harassment," Brad Sears, et al., UCLA School of Law Williams Institute; August 2024 (https://williamsinstitute.law.ucla.edu/publications/lgbt-workplace-discrimination/).

62 "Researchers find disparities in suicide risk among lesbian, gay and bisexual adults," National Institutes of Health; November 9, 2021 (https://www.nih.gov/news-events/news-releases/researchers-find-disparities-suicide-risk-among-lesbian-gay-bisexual-adults).

63 "2023 U.S. National Survey on the Mental Health of LGBTQ+ Young People," The Trevor Project; undated (https://www.thetrevorproject.org/survey-2023/).

64 "Affirmative Therapy," *Psychology Today*; undated (https://www.psychologytoday.com/us/therapy-types/affirmative-therapy#:~:text=Affirmative%20therapy%20is%20primarily%20used,homophobia%20may%20have%20influenced%20them).

65 "How to Support Your LGBTQ Grandchild," Nancy Fitzgerald, SilverSneakers; December 19, 2021 (https://www.silversneakers.com/blog/how-to-support-your-lgbtq-grandchild/).

66 "Studies Say that Gay Couples Divorce Less Frequently than Straight Couples," Faulkner Law Group; October 18, 2023 (https://www.faulknerlawgroup.com/studies-say-that-gay-couples-divorce-less-frequently-than-straight-couples/).

67 "LGBTQ People's Experiences of Workplace Discrimination and Harassment," Brad Sears, et al., UCLA School of Law Williams Institute; August 2024 (https://williamsinstitute.law.ucla.edu/publications/lgbt-workplace-discrimination/).

## PART SIX: FAMILIES

68 "Census Bureau Releases New Report on Living Arrangements of Children," United States Census Bureau; February 3, 2022 (https://www.census.gov/newsroom/press-releases/2022/living-arrangements-of-chldren.html#:~:text=3%2C%202022%20%E2%80%94%20According%20to%20a%20new,the%20children%20living%20with%20two%20parents%20l).

69 "Sociodemographic Characteristics of LGBTQ Parents in the United States," Children's Bureau Express; November 2024 (https://cbexpress.acf.hhs.gov/article/2024/november/sociodemographic-characteristics-of-lgbtq-parents-in-the-united-states/e98f46388795d210106fb848cebb3569).

70 "Kids Raised By Same-Sex Parents Fare Same As—Or Better Than—Kids Of Straight Couples, Research Finds," Robert Hart, *Forbes*; March 6, 2023 (https://www.forbes.com/sites/roberthart/2023/03/06/kids-raised-by-same-sex-parents-fare-same-as-or-better-than-kids-of-straight-couples-research-finds/)

71 "U.S. has world's highest rate of children living in single-parent households," Pew Research Center; December 12, 2019 (https://www.pewresearch.org/short-reads/2019/12/12/u-s-children-more-likely-than-children-in-other-countries-to-live-with-just-one-parent/).

72 "Child Well-Being in Single-Parent Families," The Annie E. Casey Foundation; April 6, 2024 (https://www.aecf.org/blog/child-well-being-in-single-parent-families).

73 "Family Meals and Child Academic Behavioral Outcomes," Daniel P. Miller, et al., National Institute of Health, National Library of Medicine; November 1, 2013 (https://pmc.ncbi.nlm.nih.gov/articles/PMC3498594/).

74 "The American Family Today," Pew Research Center; December 17, 2015 (https://www.pewresearch.org/social-trends/2015/12/17/1-the-american-family-today/).

75 "10 Factors to Consider Before Moving Your Elderly Parents In," Mard Naman, SeniorNavigator; April 4, 2024 (https://seniornavigator.org/article/66967/10-factors-consider-moving-your-elderly-parents).

76 "A majority of young adults in the U.S. live with their parents for the first time since the Great Depression," Pew Research Center; September 4, 2020 (https://www.pewresearch.org/short-reads/2020/09/04/a-majority-of-young-adults-in-the-u-s-live-with-their-parents-for-the-first-time-since-the-great-depression/).

77 "More Adults living with their parents," Census 2021, Office for National Statistics; May 10, 2023 (https://www.ons.gov.uk/peoplepopulationandcommunity/populationandmigration/populationestimates/articles/moreadultslivingwiththeirparents/2023-05-10).

## PART SEVEN: RELATIONSHIPS

78 "6 Relationship Resolutions for the New Year," Catherine Pearson, *New York Times*; January 1, 2025 (https://www.nytimes.com/2025/01/01/well/family/relationship-advice-resolutions-2025-new-year.html?searchResultPosition=1).

79 "Marriage rates are up, and divorce rates are down, new data shows," Madeline Holcombe, CNN Health; March 19, 2024 (https://www.cnn.com/2024/03/17/health/marriage-divorce-rates-wellness/index.html).

80 "How Much Does Divorce Cost?" RocketMoney; April 22, 2024 (https://www.rocketmoney.com/learn/investing/how-much-does-divorce-cost#:~:text=The%20average%20cost%20of%20a%20divorce%20in,and%20even%20the%20state%20they%20reside%20in.&text=Filing%20fees:%20Filing%20fees%20for%20divorce%20proceedings,a%20few%20hundred%20to%20several%20hundred%20dollars).

81 "How to Avoid Online Scams and What to Do if You Become a Victim," Tara Siegel Bernar, *New York Times*; August 15, 2024 (https://www.nytimes.com/2024/08/10/business/online-scams-advice.html?searchResultPosition=1).

82 "Killed by a scam: A father took his life after losing his savings to international criminal gangs. He's not the only one," Teele Rebane and Ivan Watson, CNN; June 20, 2024 (https://www.cnn.com/2024/06/17/asia/pig-butchering-scam-southeast-asia-dst-intl-hnk/index.html).

83 "Woman Discovers She Has Spent $1.4 Million in Possible Love Scam – Dr. Phil," *Dr. Phil*, YouTube; June 1, 2015 (https://www.youtube.com/watch?v=Ud8vm01nzMw).

84 "Marrying a Younger Woman: The Pros and Cons," Sylvia Smith, Marriage.com; March 13, 2024 (https://www.marriage.com/advice/relationship/marrying-a-younger-woman-the-pros-and-the-cons/).

85 "Rebounding Rupert's greatest fear, and, no, it's not mortality," Kerri Sackville, *Sydney Morning Herald*; March 23, 2023 (https://www.smh.com.au/lifestyle/life-and-relationships/rebounding-rupert-s-greatest-fear-and-no-it-s-not-mortality-20230322-p5cuey.html).

86 "Why Older Women Dating Younger Men Are More Satisfied," Justin J. Lehmiller, PhD, *Psychology Today*; March 23, 2023 (https://www.psychologytoday.com/us/blog/the-myths-of-sex/202303/older-women-who-date-younger-men-are-more-satisfied).

# ABOUT THE AUTHOR

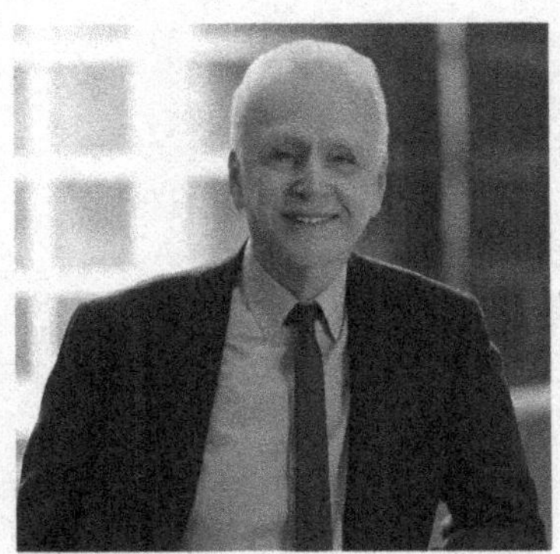

**Arnold L. Gilberg, MD, PhD**, received his bachelor's degree in political science and Doctor of Medicine degree from the University of Illinois. He interned at the Los Angeles General Medical Center. He is the last person alive trained by Franz Alexander, MD, a distinguished colleague of Sigmund Freud. His psychiatric training took place at the Cedars-Sinai Medical Center, where he was chief psychiatric resident. He also has a doctorate in psychoanalysis from the Southern California Psychoanalytic Institute.

Dr. Gilberg is a distinguished life fellow of the American Psychiatric Association, the former clinical chief of psychiatry at Cedars-Sinai Medical Center in Los Angeles, and an associate clinical professor at UCLA School of Medicine (honorary). He served for ten years under three different governors on the

Medical Board of California for LA County, and has treated thousands of patients in his Los Angeles-based practice.

Today he lives with his wife in LA, where he continues to see patients on a regular basis.